THE WONDERS
OF
QIGONG

A Chinese Exercise
For Fitness, Health, and Longevity

Compiled by

CHINA SPORTS MAGAZINE
Beijing, China

Published by

WAYFARER PUBLICATIONS
P.O. Box 26156
Los Angeles, CA 90026

Copyright © 1985 *China Sports Magazine*

Printed in the United States of America
First Printing 1985

PUBLISHED BY:
WAYFARER PUBLICATIONS
P.O. Box 26156
Los Angeles, CA 90026

Cover design by Edwin Francis

Library of Congress Catalog Card Number 82-51522
Library of Congress Cataloging in Publication Data

The Wonders of qigong.
1. Ch'i kung — Therapeutic use. 2. Ch'i kung.
I. China sports.
RM727.C54W66 1985   613'.192   85-51522

ISBN 0-935099-07-7 (pbk.)

TABLE OF CONTENTS

INTRODUCTION

Many Oriental concepts that appear strange and unbelievable to Westerners are accepted as tangible, everyday realities in China because they have been a palpable part of their culture for thousands of years. They have been experienced and validated over and over again.

Western culture questions these new realities, and rightly so, until their truth and value are proven. But it is wise to temper skepticism with an open-mindedness. Many Oriental concepts and practices have much to offer.

In the case of qigong (pronounced ch'i kung), being open and receptive can produce special benefits that the Chinese people would like to share with us in this unique mind/body discipline.

The way to access these benefits is try for ourselves the experience that the Chinese have enjoyed over the centuries. It is the goal of the book to make that possible.

Qigong is hugely popular in China today. It is estimated there are over two million practitioners. People young and old crowd into the parks in the morning to practice together. It has also been featured on television. Some teachers are reputed to have almost supernatural powers, some of which are described in this book.

The government has recognized qigong's value and set up many research institutes and sanatoriums for qigong treatment. In major cities, clinical researches on qigong are being carried out. There are qigong research organizations in Europe, the USA, Canada, Japan, and Australia. In some places, there are lectures and courses at colleges and universities.

Qigong has been practiced for many centuries to prevent and cure illness and to make the individual's daily life more useful and satisfying. Many martial artists practice qigong to enhance their power and skill.

It is best described as an energy exercise that balances and amplifies the intrinsic energy in the body. The exercise is often, but not necessarily, connected with breathing, and includes simple and sometimes complex coordinated movements of the arms and legs with the torso.

Qigong usually is done in gentle, circular and stretching movements. Sometimes it is even performed just standing, sitting or lying down with special breathing techniques so that the body can collect instead of continually disperse energy.

In China, qigong has been found to calm the nervous system by adjusting the equilibrium between excitation and inhibition. The efficiency of the respiratory system is improved, and so is the blood circulation. Different kinds of qigong methods can be used to adjust blood pressure.

The exercises promote better digestion by stimulating gastrointestinal movements and the secretion of digestive juice. They have a reputation for helping to bring a person's body weight to a normal level.

The results from the exercises are real and not especially unusual if viewed from a common sense point of view. Sometimes the results are quite dramatic, as evidenced in some of the case histories described in this book.

Some qigong experts exhibit extraordinary powers. One of these is Ma Chun, who is described in this book. Through constant practice, he developed the ability to project through his fingers and palms an outflowing energy that could cure certain diseases.

His "magic palms" emit this energy from an acupuncture point on his hand and send it into a patient's body, creating a feeling similar to when an acupuncture treatment is being given. One man with a compressed fracture of the lumbar vertebrae who had been confined to his bed in a hospital for a long time was able to leave the hospital after only 20 days of treatment.

Guo Lin, a woman now in her 70s, developed a set of exercises that cured her of cancer and restored many other seriously ill people to good health.

Take, for instance, the case of Zhou Shiyuan who had neurasthenia, gastroenteritis, hepatitis, and arthritis and had three debilitating operations, but who was able to resume a regular job within two years. A woman with oral cancer facing radiation treatment found that qigong supplemented her therapy.

In Purple Bamboo Park, Beijing, many cancer patients practice qigong to improve their health and overcome the side effects of various kinds of therapy.

A number of well-documented case histories are described in this book, which contains authoritative articles about qigong which were printed in *China Sports Magazine*, the leading English-language sports and fitness magazine in China. These articles were compiled by the editors of China Sports.

This book is published by Wayfarer Publications in order to bring qigong and its benefits to you.

The cases in this book do not suggest that qigong is a cure-all or that it alone can cure cancer or other diseases. A qualified medical authority should always be consulted first concerning an illness.

But the study of qigong does indicate that conscientious practice of these kinds of exercises will produce good health maintenance, a less stressful life, a good sense of well-being and, in some instances, extraordinarily beneficial cures from certain illnesses when combined with competent medical therapy.

The benefits from qigong do not result from any deception, self-hypnosis, or supernatural activity. Rather, it is from relaxed, enjoyable exercise that helps to balance and unblock the body's inherent energy.

After learning about the fundamentals and the benefits of qigong, try some of the simpler exercises and work your way through to the more complex.

You may even find it beneficial to isolate some of the forms of various routines and do them as individual exercises.

You will find it well worth your while to learn and practice these clearly described and easy to learn exercises that now benefit many millions of people in China.

Marvin Smalheiser
Publisher
Wayfarer Publications

FOREWORD

Over the years CHINA SPORTS has devoted much space to the exposition of qigong, a traditional form of fitness exercise whose origin can be traced back 2,000 years. The response of our readers has been most enthusiastic. Letters have kept pouring in, some confirming the salubrious effects of the exercise, others asking for more information on the subject, and many suggesting that a collection of articles be published in book form.

This is what has prompted us to present this book under the title *The Wonders of Qigong*.

The book consists of three parts. Part I provides a general description of qigong — its origin and development, contents and methods of practice, and its evaluation in the light of modern science. Part II introduces a variety of exercises, including several sophisticated forms for advanced learners as well as simple ones that can be easily mastered by beginners. Part III tells the experience both of qigong masters who have successfully applied their art to treating diseases and of ailing people who have benefited from regular practice of qigong exercises.

Thanks to its well-proven value in health-keeping and the convenient way it is practiced, qigong has aroused the interest of millions of people, not only in its native land, but in many other countries as well. The publication of this book, we hope, will help to further promote this traditional exercise for the benefit of mankind.

China Sports Magazine
Beijing
China

Wayfarer Publications publishes a newsletter on
T'ai Chi Ch'uan called T'AI CHI and
sells books and video tapes
about T'ai Chi Ch'uan and related subjects.

Information and a catalog can be obtained
by writing to:

WAYFARER PUBLICATIONS
P.O. Box 26156
Los Angeles, CA 90026

PART I

QIGONG: ITS ORIGIN AND DEVELOPMENT

By LI MEIBIN

Associate Editor-in-Chief, China Sports Magazine

Qigong (pronounced ch'i kung), which literally means "breathing exercise," has a long history in China and is a kind of traditional exercise practiced by the Chinese people to keep fit. In recent years, it has aroused the interest and attention of an increasing number of people at home and abroad.

According to the theory of Chinese medicine, qi in qigong not only means the air we breathe in, but refers as well to our inner vital energy. In modern medical terms, it means resistance to diseases, adaptability to the external environment and ability to overcome internal troubles and regain health. In traditional Chinese medicine, great importance is attached to exercise that strengthens the vital, or internal, energy.

Contents and Methods

The contents of qigong are varied, but they mainly involve the following aspects: regulation of body (posture), regulation of mind, regulation of respiration, self-massage, and movements of the limbs.

There are many schools of breathing exercises in China. Some people have classified them into five major schools, namely: medical, Confucian, Buddhist, Taoist, and wushu, or Chinese martial art. Each has its own characteristics. Medical breathing exercise aims at strengthening one's health and is good for treating and preventing diseases.

The aim of the Confucian school of breathing exercise is self-cultivation and the training of one's temperament, while the aim of Taoist breathing exercise is the cultivation of one's moral character and the seeking of longevity.

As to the Buddhist breathing exercise, which essentially involves the mind, there are two schools. One is called "Samadhi," which claims that all things in the world are illusory, and the other is called "meditation," which stresses the cultivation of the mind and the need to save all living organisms on Earth.

The wushu breathing exercise is mainly for the purpose of physical training and the improvement of health.

Though differing in purpose and method, the various schools have one thing in common — the training of the mind and the strengthening of qi (vital energy).

In ancient China, qigong was used as a means of curing diseases and improving health. When did it originate? According to the researches made by Guo Moruo, the late well-known historian and president of the Chinese Academy of Sciences, there were records of the breathing exercise in the "jin wen" (writings on bronzes) of the Zhou Dynasty (c. 1100-221 B.C.).

During the Spring and Autumn and the Warring States periods (770-221 B.C.), with the emergence of numerous thinkers and contention among a hundred schools of thought, qigong developed as never before. In the Book of Changes, semen, internal energy, and mind were regarded as the three treasures in the human body.

Daoyin, another ancient form of fitness exercise, was very popular at that time. On a cultural relic belonging to the Warring States period, the following words were carved: "Take a deep breath and sink it to 'dantian' (an acupuncture point slightly below the navel). Hold the breath there for a while and then exhale it like the sprouting grass until it goes to the top of your head. In this way, the 'yang' (masculine or positive) vital energy would go up and the 'yin' (female or negative) down. Those whose 'yang' or 'yin' vital energy goes its own way would live, otherwise they would die." This is what the ancients called daoyin and what we call qigong nowadays. This is a comparatively systematic exposition of the theory of qigong.

Many Old Treatises

Among the well-preserved sacrificial objects excavated in Tomb No. 3 at Mawangdui in Changsha, the capital of the Hunan Province, there were many medical treatises and special books about daoyin dating back to the Western Han Dynasty (206 B.C.-24 A.D.). These included painted figures of both sexes and different ages on 44 pieces of colored silk doing various daoyin movements. Some imitated the movements of the tiger, deer, bear, ape, and bird. These were later called the "wuqinxi," or "five-animal play." All these limb movements were combined with breathing. By the side of a figure with the two arms moving backward, for instance, the words "look skyward and exhale" were written.

In the book "Huang Di Neijing" ("The Yellow Emperor's Manual of Internal Medicine"),

China's earliest extant medical classic, which was written in the Warring States Period, there is a passage which reads: "One must breathe the essence of life, regulate one's respiration to preserve one's spirit and keep the muscles relaxed." In another section, it says that "those with kidney trouble can do this set of exercises in order to cure the disease. Stand with the face turned to the south in the early morning and breathe in seven times without thinking of anything."

Qigong and Wushu Combined

After the Eastern Han Dynasty (25-220 A.D.), with the introduction of Buddhism, the Indian Buddhists' yoga was combined with the ancient daoyin of our country, thereby promoting the development of qigong both in theory and practice. It is said that in the Southern and Northern Dynasties (420-589 A.D.), an eminent Indian monk came to China and set up Zen (Ch'an) Buddhism in Henan's Shaolin Monastery. He evolved a set of exercises for keeping fit, combining qigong with wushu.

From the Han Dynasty (206 B.C.-220 A.D.) to the Tang Dynasty (618-907 A.D.), qigong was widely used in medical treatment and many famous doctors were at the same time qigong masters who made great contributions to qigong therapy. Hua Tuo (?-208 A.D.), a great physician, knew how to keep in good health, and he looked as healthy and strong as a young man even in his old age. He later passed on the methods of daoyin to his disciples.

Chao Yuanfang, a famous doctor in the Sui Dynasty (581-618 A.D.), pointed out that when a man had mastered qigong he could release through his palm a kind of vital energy to cure diseases in others. Sun Simao (581-682 A.D.), another famous doctor in Chinese history, who lived for over 100 years, did some research work on medicine. In his "One Thousand Prescriptions," he expounded the theory and practice of daoyin.

By the Song Dynasty (960-1279), some Confucians, who had failed in their imperial examinations, turned to the medical profession. In their theoretical studies, however, they laid too much emphasis on the classical works and neglected practice. As a result, qigong declined and was popular only among the folk doctors. But, as luck would have it, researches on the theory of qigong were carried on in religious circles and its use was integrated with wushu.

From the Song to the Qing Dynasties (960-1911), although qigong developed greatly in practice, it was tainted with mysticism and superstition, thereby straying into a blind alley.

Since the beginning of this century, with the introduction of modern sciences, research work on qigong has been undertaken from a new angle. The useful and essential parts are selected and preserved, while the dross is discarded, and several sets of beneficial exercises for keeping fit have been compiled. One of these is Baduanjin, or Brocade Exercises in Eight Forms, which is gaining in popularity among the people.

A New Development

In recent years, due importance has been attached to the study of qigong, with heartening results. With the support of the government, many qigong research institutes and sanatoriums have been set up, making qigong more popular than ever before.

In some big Chinese cities, like Beijing and Shanghai, clinical researches on qigong are carried out, and some qigong masters are able to emit internal qi in the treatment of patients suffering from high blood pressure, neurosis, functional disease, paralysis agitans sequelae of cerebral concussion and tumors in the thyroid gland. It is also sometimes used as an anesthetic in operations.

Modern scientific instruments have been used in researches on qigong, and have detected infrared, electro-magnetic wave information, static information and magnetic information from the qi released by qigong masters. These findings will help push the study of qigong to a higher stage and contribute to the human endeavor in probing the mysteries of life.

DAOYIN: AN ANCIENT FORM OF FITNESS EXERCISE

By WANG JIAFU

Associate Professor of Sports Medicine, Hunan Medical College

Changsha, the capital of Hunan Province, is an ancient city south of the Yangtze River and was known for its flourishing metallurgical, textile and lacquer crafts as early as in the Spring and Autumn and Warring States periods (770-221 B.C.). At Mawangdui, on the city's eastern outskirts, two Han tombs were excavated in 1972-73. The ingenious structure of the tombs and the well-preserved funeral objects found in them reflect the relatively high economic level of that period.

In one of the tombs (Tomb No. 3), which belonged to a general of the Western Han Dynasty (206 B.C.-24 A.D.), large quantities of weapons as well as books on medicine were found. The latter include "Jingmai," which deals with certain vital passages in the human body, and "52 Typical Prescriptions." Most notable among the finds is a silk scroll on which were over 40 human figures with different postures drawn in black lines and painted in color. Some of the figures and explanatory Chinese characters are hardly legible.

But after intensive research, they have been identified as a series of daoyin diagrams belonging to the early Western Han Dynasty. Judging from the appearance of the figures and the descriptions of their movements as well as the names of diseases referred to, they are probably the earliest existing diagrams of exercises for promoting health and curing diseases. They testify to the rich experiences gained by the Chinese people through age-long struggles against ailments and illnesses of one kind or another.

Breathing and Movement Are Combined

Daoyin is an ancient method of health building that combines regulated breathing with body movements. It was recorded in "Neijing" over 2,000 years ago. During the latter period of the Eastern Han Dynasty (25-220 A.D.), the celebrated physician Hua Tuo made a thorough study of the traditional theories and practice of daoyin, and on this basis created a set of exercises called wuqinxi (pronounced woo chin see).

Literally meaning five-animal play, it consisted of movements mimicking those of a tiger thrusting forward its foreleg, a deer craning and turning its neck, a bear crouching and then standing erect, an ape hopping on its toes, a bird soaring with outspread wings, and so forth. Bringing out to the full the characteristic features of daoyin, the wuqinxi exercises helped to limber up the muscles and joints and proved its value in health protection and in the treatment of diseases. As these exercises were easy to learn, they caught on very quickly.

Books and diagrams about daoyin appeared in growing numbers in the Western Jin Dynasty (266-316 A.D.). By the time of the Sui and Tang dynasties (581-907 A.D.) daoyin had branched out into other forms of fitness exercises, such as the popular baduanjin and taijiquan. Numerous works and diagrams dealing with them were published. All of these provided useful background information for the study of the daoyin paintings unearthed from Tomb No. 3 at Mawangdui.

The figures in these paintings are of both sexes and different ages, dressed in different attire and doing various movements, mostly bare-handed and occasionally with weapons. Traces of these movements are found in setting-up exercises which spread among the people in later periods.

The daoyin exercises are good for all the joints in the human body and at the same time lay particular stress on strengthening the shoulders, the waist, the knees, and the respiratory organs. The methods of training and the principles involved are basically the same as those expounded in modern medical literature.

The following are drawings of descriptions of some of the exercises shown on the ancient silk scroll found at Changsha.

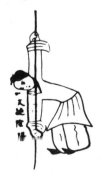

Figure 1

Bend and turn the body with
the support of a pole.

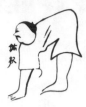

Figure 2

Bend forward at the waist, with the palms touching the floor, and draw up the chin as much as possible.

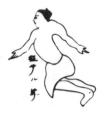

Figure 3

Kneel on the floor and turn the trunk.

Figure 4

Sit on the floor and turn the trunk.

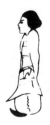

Figure 5

Keep both hands hanging naturally and bend the legs slightly at the knees.

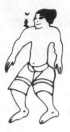

Figure 6

Stand with the knees slightly bent and hands slightly extended outward.

The exercises for strengthening the muscles of the lower limbs and curing ailments in the knee joints as shown in Figs. 5 and 6, are similar to those practiced today. They testify to a fairly deep knowledge of the anatomy of the lower limbs and an elementary understanding of the laws of their movements.

In the case of upper limb movements, breathing exercise goes hand in hand with the exercise of the shoulder joints to improve the functions of the heart and lungs.

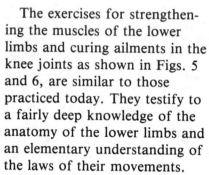

Figure 7

Stand erect and raise both arms shoulder high sideways, with the palms turned upward and chest expanded.

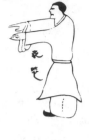

Figure 8

Stand erect, with both arms stretched forward shoulder high and the palms facing downward.

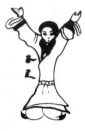

Figure 9

Stand erect and raise both arms upward and outward like a bird spreading its wings.

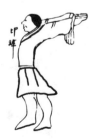

Figure 10

Stand erect and raise both hands upward and backward while keeping the chest out and taking a deep breath.

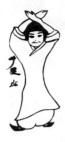

Figure 11

Stand erect, raise both hands and cross them overhead.

With the help of modern medical knowledge, we can make use of the daoyin movements in a scientific way and work out setting-up or remedial exercises suitable for various age groups of both sexes and for strengthening different parts of the body.

The unearthed daoyin diagrams are a new discovery of ancient Chinese medical literature. They provide valuable material for the further study of the origin and development of this unique method of therapy.

The restored Western Han painting on daoyin exercises, which are the earliest forms of what we call qigong today.

马王堆三号汉墓出土导引图复原图

REVEALING THE MYSTERY OF LIFE

By SHU CHI

Researcher, China Sports History Committee

The spectators gaped with astonishment as they watched a visiting performer thrust a spear against his throat. Another performer supported himself at the belly with the prong of a fork. A third received hard blows on a sword placed on his own chest and then, lying on a nailed board, he took the impact of hammer blows that would smash the stone slab placed over his body.

The performances given by three Chinese qigong masters who toured Luxembourg, Italy, Belgium, France, and Romania in the winter of 1979, created nothing short of a sensation.

In Luxembourg, there was such a big turnout at one show that there were not enough seats although they had been provisionally increased to twice the usual number. In Belgium, many football fans chose to attend a qigong exhibition rather than an international match against West Germany. And curious Italian spectators swarmed into the arena to pick up bits of bricks that had been piled on the head of a performer and shattered with a hammer, or to ask for the performers' autographs.

Many foreigners who had watched the incredible feats admired qigong as a gem in the treasure house of human endeavors and suggested that it should be carefully studied.

Daoyin an Ancient Therapeutic Technique

According to archeological finds, qigong was widely used as a therapeutic means by our ancestors around 400 B.C., having evolved from yet older forms of breathing exercises such as daoyin, tuna (exhalation and inhalation), neiquan (introversion), and jingzuo (meditation). Stories about qigong feats by wushu masters abound in history books.

For instance, "Hitting the bare chest with the blade of a sword" was recorded during the Warring States period (475-221 B.C.) and is quite similar to the modern version. During the reign of Dezong (780-805 A.D.) in the Tang Dynasty, there was a man of unusual strength named Wang Jie in Changan, now Xian, the capital of Shaansi Province.

While lying on the ground, he could bear the weight of a group of musicians playing on a platform supported by a seven-meter-long wooden pillar erected on top of a millstone placed on his body. Aspects of his feat can be found in some of the performances given by individuals today.

Although there were numerous varieties of qigong and many different methods of training, none can be done without the exercise of "yi" (mental activity), and qi, or the "flow of vitality," which includes but is not limited to breathing. Yi plays the leading role over qi.

In other words, the accumulation, circulation, and release of a man's vital energy is controlled and regulated by the mind. Exercising the control power of his mind, a qigong master is able to perform marvelous feats by mustering all his vital energy and concentrating it in a certain part of his body for the release of a tremendous explosive strength.

But what exactly do we mean by qi? And how is it generated, circulated, and released?

While it is common knowledge that man's will can react upon the objective world, few people are able to explain why it plays such a significant role in regulating and controlling the functions of his own body. The widespread practice of qigong in ancient times provided rich perceptual knowledge which should have promoted theoretical research in this sphere.

Unfortunately, in those days, qigong was shrouded in mystery owing to the influence of religion and was likewise mystified in classical novels, so that it was looked upon superstitiously and as quackery and was, therefore, given little serious attention.

Significant Research Started in 1949

Serious research in this field began only after the founding of New China in 1949. Early in the 1960s, medical researchers in Shanghai made a preliminary study of the physiological aspects of qigong.

Examinations of practitioners in a relaxed and tranquil state showed a slowing down of heart rates, a decreased frequency of respiration and a marked reduction of oxygen consumption — in some cases falling to 70 percent of the normal level, or lower than the amount consumed by a sleeping man. All these were considered to be indications of energy accumulation in the human body, a peculiar physiological phenomenon which aroused interest in scientific circles.

In November 1977, scientists at the Atomic Nucleus Research Institute of the Academy of Sciences of China detected low-frequency modulated infrared radiation in the waiqi (outflowing energy) released from the hands of Lin Housheng, a qigong master at the Institute of Traditional Chinese Medicine.

As we know, infrared radiation — a kind of electromagnetic wave — can be released by any human body. Ordinarily, however, such radiation is negligible and shows an almost straight line on the recorder, whereas in Lin's case the infrared radiation emitted stronger signals. Thus, qi, invisible as it is to the naked eye, was clinically identified as a form of matter.

A similar discovery was later made with qigong practitioner Zhao Guang by the Beijing Research Institute of Traditional Chinese Medicine. At the moment of the emission of energy, a 20 percent increase in micro-circulation at Zhao's fingertips was recorded, showing that the release of signals was effected at the expense of energy loss from his body.

A Strong Pulse Signal 50 mm Above His Head

As training methods vary, the nature of waiqi released by practitioners also varies from case to case. For example, Liu Jinrong bent a steel ruler (4 mm thick, 40 mm wide and 700 mm long) after twice slapping it hard on his ribs. He then straightened it with another two forceful strokes on his head.

As he continued to focus his radiation energy, a strong pulse signal of static electricity was detected at a point 50 mm above his head. A magnetic field was also noted whose unusual strength exceeded the range of the recorder, setting it buzzing with a loud noise and breaking the recording pen.

Zhao Wei, another practitioner, emitted a different kind of waiqi via the tips of his index and middle fingers that could shake a hanging thread or stir up dust from a distance of one meter. With a swish of his two fingers above his thigh, there instantly appeared on it a reddish stripe about one centimeter wide as if it were caused by the slash of a whip.

Diagnostic tests showed that his waiqi was neither infrared radiation nor static electricity. It was probably an ejection of some other substance that has yet to be identified. Some think it might be a current of micro-particles, some suggest a thermodynamic flow, while others try to define it as something similar to but not exactly the same as an air current. There is much controversy and no definite conclusion has been reached as yet.

Some Qigong Masters Can Cure Certain Ailments

According to clinical experiments by the Shanghai Research Institute of Traditional Chinese Medicine and other bodies, waiqi released by qigong masters can help cure some ailments by inducing certain unknown physiological and biochemical effects in the patient. In the light of these experiments, some research units in cooperation with hospitals have trial-produced bionic instruments for therapeutic use, with satisfactory results.

During the last decade and more, qigong has gained a great deal of headway outside its native country, often under the name of "Chinese yoga," although actually it is quite different from yoga exercises as practiced by Buddhists in India.

According to statistics, there are now about two million qigong followers in various parts of the world, with special research organizations having been set up in some European countries, the USA, Canada, Japan and Australia. In some places, qigong lectures and courses are given at colleges and universities. Academic meetings have been held to probe the secrets of this art.

Far from being illusion or superstition, qigong is a phenomenon that falls within the province of the life sciences. The discovery of its unique signals in the air has not only opened new vistas in the research of modern medical science, but is also highly significant to the study of biomedical and bionic problems.

With scientists all over the world joining their efforts to promote this traditional Chinese exercise, it will prove ever more fully its value in helping to reveal the mystery of life.

NEW PROBLEMS IN LIFE SCIENCE

By LI YINGBO

An Acoustics Researcher at the Acoustics Institute of the Chinese Academy of Sciences

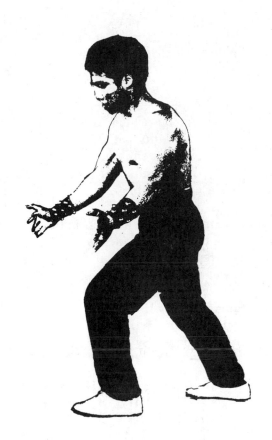

After watching the incredible performances by a qigong master who can bear enormous weights or withstand hard blows on his body, or smash a stone slab with a blow of his palm, or bend a steel ruler by slapping it hard on his chest, many people in and out of China ask:

What makes qigong practitioners' muscles harder than granite? What exactly is the qi or breath in qigong and how is it consciously directed to a certain part of the human body? Is there anything extraordinary about a qigong master's physiology?

Questions like these have aroused growing interest among scientific circles.

In June 1979, using an infrasonic detector designed and made by ourselves, we took some measurements on two qigong masters and some patients under qigong treatment. Our primary discoveries were as follows.

1. Pulse

Attached to the artery of a qigong master's right wrist, our infrasonic receiver recorded his pulse waves (See Fig. 1), which showed marked changes in both frequency and amplitude when he practiced qigong.

2. Muscle oscillations

As indicated by a probe attached to qigong master Hou Shuying's arm where he had directed his qi, his muscles were in high tension, oscillating with an amplitude about 50 times greater than that of an ordinary person simulating his movements. The other qigong master's muscles under the same test showed oscillations with both low frequencies of less than one hertz and high frequencies of 11-12 hertz, lasting quite a long while.

3. Patient under qigong treatment

The probe was fixed on an artery in the in-step of a patient suffering from protrusion of intervertebral discs. As Hou concentrated his qi in his fingertips, which produced therapeutic effects on certain acupuncture points on the patient's

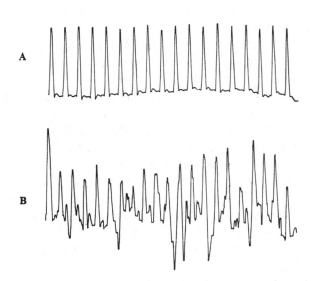

Fig. 1 Hou Shuying's pulse waves —

A. Taken before his *qigong* exercise.
B. Taken when he was practicing *qigong*.

body, marked changes were recorded in his pulse waves after two treatments, as shown in Figs. 2-3.

4. Temperature of Hou's "radioactive" palm

With the help of our highly sensitive infrasonic detector, we observed a rapid accumulation of heat in Hou's palm when he practiced qigong exercises. Within five minutes, the temperature of his "radioactive" palm was found to have risen to 38.6 degrees centigrade, or 101.48 degrees fahrenheit.

Such initial experiments have revealed some interesting phenomena which need to be further studied. What accounts for the changes in pulse waves shown by both the qigong master and the patient? Why is it possible for a qigong master to concentrate a considerable amount of heat in his palm in a few minutes?

I think we may find the answers in the theories of traditional Chinese medicine, which attach great importance to feeling the pulse as a diagnostic means, rather than in the physiological theories of the Western school, which regard the pulse merely as the regular beating in the arteries caused by the contraction of the heart.

The effect produced by a "radioactive" palm on acupuncture points is even more puzzling, since anatomically no satisfactory explanation has ever been given as to what are acupuncture points and what is jingluo, the passages along which the acupuncture points are supposed to be distributed.

However, one cannot deny the sensations caused by needles inserted into these points and conducted along the jingluo passages. In recent years, traditional Chinese medical theories have aroused increasing attention in the medical world and more phenomena of life must be approached from the traditional Chinese medical point of view, which regards the human body as an organic whole.

In the past, however, qigong therapy and traditional Chinese medicine in general were dismissed as unscientific, superstitious or witchcraft-like. This was most unfair. As an independent medical system, formed over thousands of years, they have proved their worth in preserving health and curing diseases.

We should not deny their scientific value simply because we are unable to explain them in the light of modern scientific theories, still less pronounce them to be unscientific just because we know too little about them. Rather, we should carry out deep-going research and place our newly found knowledge at the service of mankind.

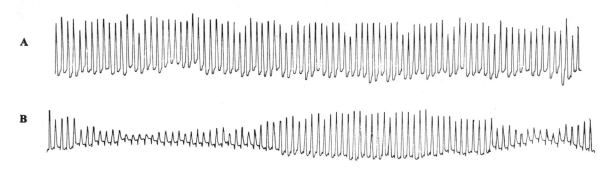

Fig. 2 The patient's pulse waves —

    A. Taken before his first treatment by Hou Shuying.
    B. Taken after the first treatment.

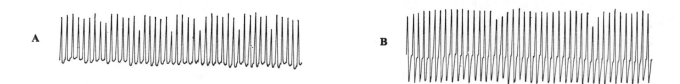

Fig. 3 The patient's pulse waves —

    A. Taken before his second treatment by Hou.
    B. Taken after the second treatment.

PART II

QIGONG: BREATHING EXERCISES

By SHI FU

Researcher, China National Qigong Society

The Chinese word qi literally means air. In traditional Chinese medicine, it refers to a person's vital energy, or "yuan qi," including but not limited to the air one breathes in. Qigong is actually a kind of breathing exercise aimed at stimulatng a person's vital energy so as to strengthen his immunity to diseases, adaptability to the external environment, and ability to repair internal damage.

Traditional Chinese medicine holds that a person full of yuan qi will enjoy good health. Of course, qigong is not a panacea for all ailments and maladies. It must be used in conjunction with other forms of exercise and therapy in order to effect a cure. To a great extent, gongfu (called kung-fu in the West) relies on the mastery of qigong techniques for the attainment of mental and physical harmony.

All forms of qigong involve three essential aspects: regulation of body position, regulation of respiration and regulation of the mind. These three aspects interact on each other. A qigong performer must strive to grasp their essentials in order to improve his health and resistance to disease.

Of the many qigong exercises, the following three forms are used most often: Relaxation exercise; Strengthening exercise; and Inward Training exercise.

Relaxation Exercise

This form is fairly easy to learn and has proved effective in varying degrees in treating some chronic diseases.

Body position:

Lie flat on your back (Fig. 1), head on pillow, arms laid comfortably by the sides, legs extended naturally, eyes and mouth slightly closed, teeth slightly clenched, and the tip of the tongue touching the hard palate.

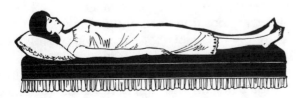

Fig. 1.

Respiration:

Breathe normally through the nose — regularly, slowly, evenly, and quietly. Contemplate the word "calm" when inhaling and the word "relax" when exhaling. Relax part of your body at each respiration, in the order of head, arms, hands, chest, abdomen, back, the small of the back, buttocks, legs, and feet. After the muscles of the whole body are relaxed, meditate on relaxing your blood vessels, nerves and viscera.

Frequency and duration of training:

Individual fitness levels will be the primary determining factor. In general, a convalescent ordered a complete rest can exercise three or four times a day, each time lasting 20 to 30 minutes. A person working part or full time can exercise once or twice a day, each time lasting 30 minutes. There is no definite length for a course of treatment. It usually takes two or three months, or even longer, to achieve noticeable effects.

Strengthening Exercise

This form of exercise can be applied to cases of neurasthenia, hypertension, heart trouble, and pulmonary emphysema. Emphasis is placed on attaining a state of tranquility rather than on regulation of the respiration.

Body positions:

Normal sitting position (Fig. 2). Sit erect on a

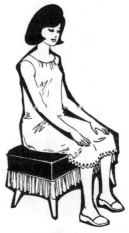

Fig. 2.

square stool with feet flat on the ground, legs shoulder-width apart at the knees, which are flexed at 90 degrees. The thighs are at right angles to the trunk, palms resting in a relaxed manner on the knees, elbows naturally bent, shoulders down, chin slightly withdrawn, chest in, and eyes, mouth and tongue kept in the same positions as in the Relaxation exercise.

Cross-legged sitting position (Fig. 3). Sit on a cushion, either with one leg folded over the other, or with both feet tucked under the legs and both knees off the cushion. Keep buttocks slightly protruding, head erect, back straight, shoulders down, chin slightly withdrawn, and chest held in.

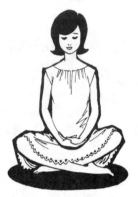

Fig. 3.

Place hands below the navel or over the small of the abdomen, with thumbs locked and palms facing upward. For eyes, mouth, and tongue follow the same instructions as in the Relaxation exercise.

Standing position (Fig. 4). Stand with feet shoulder-width apart and slightly turned in, knees

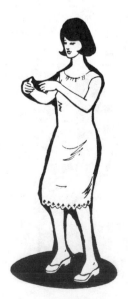

Fig. 4.

slightly bent, back straight, chest in, arms raised as if encircling a big tree. The hands are at shoulder level. The elbows are lowered, and the fingers form a circle as if clutching a ball.

Respiration:

Natural breathing: Breathe through the nose as in the Relaxation exercise.

Abdominal breathing: Inflate the abdomen naturally while inhaling and deflate it while exhaling. With no pause between inspiration and expiration, breathing should gradually be deepened to reach six to eight full cycles per minute. This must be done naturally without forcing a deep breath.

Attainment of tranquility:

Focus your attention on the abdomen — this is the basis of the Strengthening exercise. In the initial stages of training, it may be achieved in the following way:

— Count from 1 to 10 as you breathe, one number for each cycle of respiration. Begin over again if distractions cause your mind to wander. Repeat the 1 to 10 count several times in succession.

— Purge your mind of all distracting thoughts and let it follow the rise and fall of your abdomen naturally while breathing.

— Bring your attention to a point about 5 cm below the navel, allowing it to hover there without overstraining your mind. Try again if your mind wanders.

Inward Training Exercise

This is particularly suitable to the individual suffering from duodenal ulcers, hepatitis, constipation, or ptosis of the stomach. Emphasis is placed on breathing.

Body positions:

Normal sitting position as in the Strengthening exercise.

Supine position as in the Relaxation exercise.

Side lying position as in Fig. 5. Lie on your side (usually on the right) with the head slightly forward, right arm bent and resting on the pillow while the left arm is extended naturally, hand on hip with palm downward. Left leg on the right, both legs slightly bent.

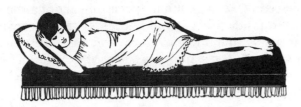

Fig. 5.

Other positions may also be adopted, provided they are natural and comfortable.

Respiration:

Breathe abdominally through the nose — inhale, exhale, pause (i.e. stop breathing) for 3-7 seconds, inhale, exhale, pause . . . repeat. During each pause, raise your tongue and meditate before dropping your tongue and inhaling again.

As you meditate, say something meaningful to yourself silently, such as "Be calm," "Relax," and "It's good to be calm and relax." Each syllable should last for a second.

Progressively lengthen the pauses by saying more words. Do not hold your breath with effort, nor try to hold it in your chest or throat. Just stop breathing and focus your attention on the region of the navel.

The physiological functions of the pauses require further investigation, but preliminary studies suggest that these respiratory exercises bring about cyclic changes in internal abdominal pressure, which activate blood circulation in the abdomen and promote gastrointestinal peristalsis.

Attainment of tranquility:

Tranquility is gradually acquired by coordinating respiration with contemplation of selected words, which helps concentration and keeps the mind from wandering.

	Stage I (1st week)	Stage II (2nd-4th weeks)	Stage III (5th week and beyond)
Body position	Normal sitting position (or supine position for those in delicate health)	Normal or cross-legged sitting position	Sitting or standing position (the latter for stronger trainees)
Respiration	From natural to slightly deep breathing	Natural deep breathing (abdominal)	
Attainment of tranquility	Count respirations or just follow them mentally	Follow respirations mentally or concentrate on a point 5 cm below navel	Concentrate on a point 5 cm below navel
Frequency & duration	3-4 times daily, each time 15-20 min.	3-4 times daily, each time 30 min.	3-4 times daily, each time 30-45 min.
Requirements	1) Correct position; 2) Regulated breathing; 3) Freedom from distractions	1) Deep breathing down to diaphragm; 2) Initial tranquility; 3) Training becomes habitual	1) Regular, deep, even breathing: 2) Complete tranquility; 3) Noticeable benefits motivate further training

How Does Qigong Cure Diseases?

Qigong has proved effective in treating certain chronic disorders and, as indicated by recent experience in China, is particularly helpful to sufferers from stomach and duodenal ulcers, ptosis of the stomach, habitual constipation, neurasthenia, and high blood pressure.

The qigong works three ways.

First, it helps restore vitality. By inducing a state of tranquility, qigong allows the body to restore vital energy, build up disease resistance, and alleviate functional disorders.

Physiological experiments show that when a person is in a tranquil state induced by qigong exercise, his cerebral cortex is in an inhibited state, which allays the over-excitation of cortical cells that may result in functional disorders. This may explain why qigong has proved beneficial in the treatment of neurasthenia, hypertension and gastric ulcers, which are all closely connected with the nervous system.

Secondly, it helps conserve energy. Experimental findings indicate that in the course of doing qigong exercises oxygen consumption is reduced by 30.7 percent and energy metabolism by 20 percent. Conservation of energy is a probable factor, contributing to the effect of qigong in bringing the chronically ill back to health.

Thirdly, it massages the abdominal cavity. Qigong, particularly the Inward Training exercise, produces a massaging effect on the abdominal cavity by virtue of the mechanical action of breathing, with the diaphragm moving up and down at a much larger range than usual.

Such a massaging effect promotes gastro-intestinal peristalsis, reduces the extravasated blood in the abdomen and aids digestion and absorption. This is why one who practices qigong has a sharpened appetite and puts on weight — and also why qigong can cure habitual constipation and ptosis of the stomach.

How to Practice Qigong

To benefit from qigong exercises, the following principles should be observed:

1. Relax, keep calm, and remain at ease. First of all, relax your body. Don't shrug your shoulders or throw out your chest. Don't strain yourself to maintain your posture. Always make yourself comfortable. All muscles must be relaxed, especially those of the lower abdomen. Clothes and waistbelt should be loose.

Second, set your mind at ease and adopt a cheerful attitude, free from all cares and worries. Regulate your breathing after initial relaxation is attained. It is usually in the stage of exhalation that you can feel yourself mentally and physically relaxed.

Tranquility is attained by focusing your attention on the exercise, banishing all other thoughts from your mind, and avoiding as much as possible such external stimuli as sound and light.

Then you find yourself in such a state of perfect calm that you are unconscious even of your own body weight. You may feel irritated at being unable to concentrate in the beginning. This is quite natural. Tell yourself to calm down and be confident and patient. Persistent practice will surely bring steady progress.

2. Coordinate meditation with respiration. In qigong exercises, respiration must be guided by meditation. In other words, conscious efforts must be made to regulate the rhythm of breathing, thereby directing the flow of vital energy to various parts of the body.

While the key to meditation lies in tranquility, respiration is never satisfactory unless it is "fine, deep, long, slow, stable, leisurely and uniform." Both the Strengthening exercise and Relaxation exercise emphasize meditation, while the Inward Training exercise emphasizes respiration. But in any case meditation and respiration must be coordinated.

3. Combine motion with stillness. As qigong calls for stillness and little motion, it should be supplemented with some active exercises for better therapeutic results. Active exercises should come after qigong exercises — in other words, motion after stillness.

4. Go step by step. Qigong is an art that can be perfected only through long disciplined practice. Start with the easier methods with regard to body position, breathing, and the attainment of tranquility. Each training period lasts 15-20 minutes in the beginning and may be gradually lengthened as time goes on.

Here are some further points for attention:

1. About 15 minutes prior to a qigong exercise, stop reading and all other mental work, go to the toilet if necessary, and get ready for training.

2. Don't stand up abruptly after the exercise. Massage your face with both hands and rub your eyes gently and then stand up slowly and stretch your limbs.

3. If you are short of breath or feel irritated while doing the exercise, this may be due to inappropriate posture or method of breathing, a bad frame of mind, lack of interest in exercising, or distraction. Find out the cause and correct it.

4. If you feel dizzy or get a headache, this may be due to breathing with too much effort, impatience for quick results, or ill humor. Find out the cause and correct it.

5. Do not train on an empty or full stomach.

6. Suspend training when you are too tired or have a fever, diarrhea or a bad cold.

Prevention of Side Effects

Generally speaking, no side effects are felt in the three forms of exercise provided they are properly done. However, they do occur to beginners who are not used to the body positions and methods of breathing and meditation as required in the exercises, and who are technically not proficient enough. But these side effects can easily be prevented or overcome.

(A) Side effects in body position

1. A stiff back after sitting for a long time. This is either because you are not used to sitting that way or because of an incorrect position. To avoid this trouble, start from the supine position and gradually try the sitting position, or change to the supine position when you feel tired from sitting, or simply shorten the time of sitting.

2. Numbness in the legs while sitting in the cross-legged position. This may be prevented by limbering up your legs before sitting. If numbness still occurs, massage your legs or change their positions, or stand up and move about a little and then sit down again.

(B) Side effects in respiration

1. Difficulty in breathing and restlessness, usually caused by forced deep breathing. Take a short walk in the room and calm yourself before resettling to the meditation.

2. Shortness of breath or a stitch in the side. This usually happens when you breathe too hard or try to hold your breath too long, or try to "trap" it in the chest or throat. Symptoms will disappear once these faults are overcome.

(C) Side effects in meditation

1. Lethargy. In most cases, this occurs when you are lying down or when you are mentally exhausted. You may feel better if you sit up or gaze at the tip of your nose with half-closed eyes. Don't do qigong exercises when you are over-tired. To prevent drowsiness, which is quite common with beginners, sip some hot tea and take a short walk before sitting down for meditation.

2. Extraordinary sensations. Sometimes, while deep in a state of tranquility, you may feel numbness, itchiness, pins and needles, or a burning heat in the skin or muscles of some parts of your body. By concentrating your meditation on the small of the abdomen and refraining from breathing too deeply, these symptoms will soon disappear.

(D) Other side effects

1. Palpitation of the heart. This usually happens when, in a state of tranquility, you breathe too deeply, or hold your breath too long, or are too nervous. Find out the cause and correct it.

2. A throbbing sensation about the temple over the pillow. Remedy: Change your head position and relieve the pressure on the ear.

BADUANJIN: "BROCADE" EXERCISES IN EIGHT FORMS

Baduanjin is a set of fitness exercises that has enjoyed great popularity since time immemorial. It requires the coordination between body and limb movements on the one hand and breathing and mental activity on the other. It has much in common with the traditional daoyin methods.

"Baduan" means "eight sections" and "jin" means "brocade," which indicates a symbol of beauty. In the course of its development, there have emerged many different versions of baduanjin. Here we have chosen two sets for your practice.

The set under Part I was devised by Zhong Li in the Tang Dynasty (618-907 A.D.) and rearranged by Li Shixin, a physical education lecturer at Beijing University. The set under Part II was compiled by Zhuo Dahong, associate professor at Zhongshan Medical College, Guangzhou, on the basis of different versions.

PART I

Form 1   Hold Kunlun Mountains with Both Hands

Loosen your belt and garment. Sit upright, cross-legged, right calf crossing over left calf and both soles facing obliquely upward. Relax your whole body. Concentrate your mind, eyes looking straight ahead.

Knock your upper teeth lightly with the lower ones 36 times, with tip of tongue touching hard palate, and then pause for a little while. When your mouth is full of saliva, swallow it in three parts with a gurgling sound.

Then cover your ears with palms, fingers spread out like a fan. The little finger side of the hand faces upward. Place forefinger on middle finger and tap it on the back of the head 24 times. Take a deep breath, inhaling and exhaling lightly and evenly (Fig. 1).

Form 2   Shake the Heavenly Pillar

Sit upright, cross-legged, right calf crossing over left calf, both soles facing obliquely upward. Place right palm on left palm above navel, thumb side of right hand facing inside and that of left hand facing forward, all fingers slightly bent.

Turn head back to the left, eyes looking backward as far as possible for one or two seconds (Fig. 2). Then turn head back to the right, reversing the position of the palms with a friction. Do this exercise 24 times. Keep torso erect when you turn your head.

Form 3   Raise Arms

Sit upright with palms resting on bent knees, right calf crossing over left calf, both soles facing obliquely upward and eyes looking straight ahead. Clench hands loosely and raise them overhead past ears, as if you were hanging them from a horizontal bar (Fig. 3).

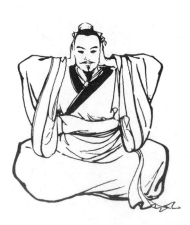

Fig 1

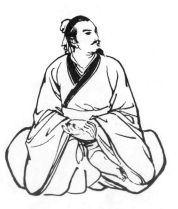

Fig 2

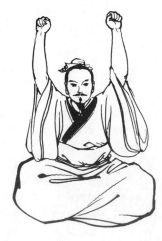

Fig 3

Stir up your tongue 36 times to produce saliva, which you swallow in three mouthfuls. Close your eyes and imagine that your heart is kindled by a torch and the flame spreads gradually to the whole body. Return palms to knees.

Form 4   Rub Lower Back

Strip yourself to waist and sit upright with right calf crossing over left calf, soles facing obliquely upward. Rub palms against each other until they are warm and place them akimbo, thumbs pointing forward and four fingers pointing obliquely downward (Fig. 4).

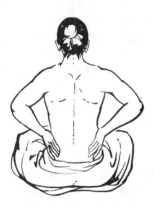

Fig 4

Rub them up and down 36 times or more against both sides of spinal cord. Put on your garment and place left palm below navel, right palm on back of left hand. Breathe lightly and imagine that the flame in your heart spreads down to the region under navel so that you feel warm all over.

Form 5   Turn Torso to One Side

Sit as you do in Form 4, right hand on hip and left palm on abdomen above navel, eyes looking straight ahead. Turn left shoulder forward and right shoulder backward and then

return to original position. Do this exercise 36 times, turning head together with shoulder (Fig. 5).

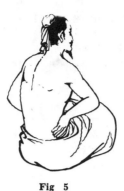

Fig 5

Form 6   Turn Torso to Both Sides

Sit as you do in Form 4. Turn left shoulder backward and then the other way around. Place both hands on hips. Do these movements 36 times, increasing degrees of rotation gradually (Fig. 6).

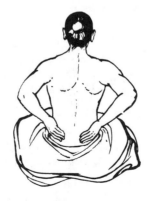

Fig 6

Place left palm on lower part of abdomen, with right palm on back of left hand. Close your eyes lightly and imagine that a flame spreads from lower part of abdomen up to the waist, through the space between the shoulder blades, and to the top of the head.

Stretch legs forward, toes pointing up and muscles

relaxed. Close your mouth slightly and take three deep breaths slowly through your nose.

Form 7   Prop Up Sky with Fingers Interlocked

Sit upright on bent legs, right calf crossing over left calf, both soles facing obliquely upward. Hands interlocked rest against abdomen, palms facing up, the little finger side of the hands touching body.

Look straight ahead. Raise palms first to chest level and then, with arms rotated internally, to overhead position. Palms face up (Fig. 7).

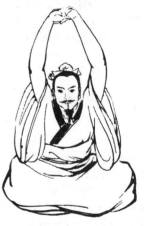

Fig 7

Then return palms to front of abdomen. Do these movements nine times, inhaling when you raise palms and exhaling when you bring them down.

Form 8   Pull Toes with Both Hands

Sit upright with legs stretched forward, feet shoulder-width apart. Place palms on floor at both sides, thumbs touching body and fingers pointing forward. Look straight ahead.

Bend forward, hold the ball and toes of one foot with both hands, pulling them back as

29

you push foot forward. Do the same with the other foot. Look at the foot in action. Do these movements 12 times, taking a deep breath slowly each time (Fig. 8).

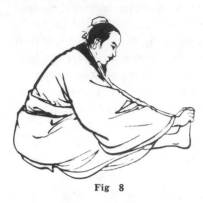

Fig 8

Sit quietly for a while with eyes and mouth slightly closed. Stir up your tongue to produce saliva, which you swallow quickly. Do these movements six times. Then shrug your shoulders and twist your waist. Relax your whole body.

This set of exercises may be practiced both morning and evening. Persistent practice will clear up the jingluo system — channels through which vital energy circulates. It will sharpen your appetite, make you sleep soundly and feel comfortable, and increase your immunity to disease.

PART II

Form 1   Prop Up the Sky with Fingers Interlocked

Starting Position: Stand at attention with heels together or feet shoulder-width apart, toes pressing against floor and arches lifted. Arms hang naturally at both sides.

Put tip of tongue lightly against hard palate, and breathe with your nose. Look straight ahead and relax all bone joints. Keep this stance for a while with concentration (Fig. 1).

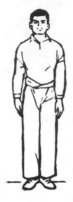

Fig 1

Movements:

A. Raise arms slowly overhead from both sides and interlock fingers overhead, with palms turned up as if to prop up the sky. Lift heels at the same time (Fig. 2).

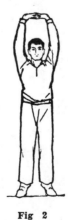

Fig 2

B. Return to starting position.

Repeat these movements many times. You may coordinate them with respiration, inhaling when you raise arms and exhaling when you put them down. This

exercise helps you to expand lungs and relieve fatigue. It also strengthens the muscles and bones of your back and helps to correct hunchback and inward-drawn shoulders. It activates your muscles and internal organs in preparation for the forms that follow.

Form 2   Draw the Bow on Both Sides

Starting Position: Stand at attention.

Movements:

A. Take a sidestep with left foot and bend both legs to form a "horse-ride step." Cross arms in front of chest, right arm on the outside. Draw left arm to the left side, with forefinger pointing up, thumb set apart and other fingers bent.

Turn head to the left to look at left forefinger. At the same time, clench right hand and draw it to the right, arm bent at shoulder level, as if you were drawing a bow (Fig. 3).

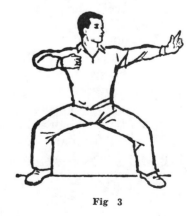

Fig 3

B. Return to starting position.

C. Repeat A, reversing "right" and "left."

D. Return to starting position.

Repeat these movements many times. You may coordinate them with respiration, inhaling when you draw your arms sideways and exhaling when you return to the starting position. This exercise helps you to strengthen the muscles of the chest, arms and shoulders. It improves respiratory and circulatory functions.

Form 3   Raise Single Arm

Starting Position: Stand at attention with heels together or feet shoulder-width apart, arms hanging naturally at both sides.

Movements:

A. Raise right hand overhead, palm turned up and fingers held together and pointing leftward. At the same time, press left hand down, fingers pointing forward (Fig. 4).

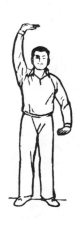

Fig 4

B. Return to starting position.

C. Repeat A, reversing "right" and "left."

D. Return to starting position.

Repeat these movements many times. You may coordinate them with respiration, inhaling when you raise one hand and press down the other and exhaling when you return to the starting position.

This exercise helps you to activate internal organs and prevent gastrointestinal disorders.

Form 4   Turn Head to Look Back

Starting Position: Stand at attention with palms pressed tightly against thighs.

Movements:

A. Turn head slowly to the left to look back (Fig. 5).

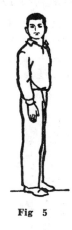

Fig 5

B. Return to starting position.

C. Turn head slowly to the right to look back.

D. Return to starting position.

Repeat these movements many times. You may coordinate them with respiration, inhaling when you turn your head and exhaling when you return to the starting position.

This exercise helps you to strengthen the muscles around the eyeballs, and to toughen neck muscles to prevent cervico-vertebral ailments. It helps to stimulate blood circulation in the head to get rid of weariness and dizziness and other functional disturbances in the central nervous system. It is particularly beneficial to sufferers of hypertension and arteriosclerosis.

Form 5   Sway Head and Buttocks

Starting Position: Stand with feet about three foot-lengths apart and bend knees to form a horse-ride step, palms on thighs and thumbs pointing backward.

Movements:

A. Lower head and bend trunk forward and then sway them to left side. At the same time, sway buttocks to the right, aiding the movement by properly stretching out left leg and hip. You may move hands a bit with the trunk movement (Fig. 6).

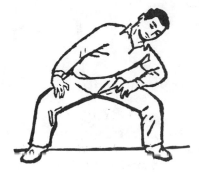

Fig 6

B. Return to starting position.

C. Repeat A, reversing "right" and "left."

D. Return to starting position.

Repeat these movements many times. You may coordinate them with respiration, inhaling when you sway trunk to either side and exhaling when you return to starting position.

This exercise helps you, to use a term of traditional Chinese medicine, "to rid the heart of fire," which means removing overstrain in the nervous system caused by physical over-exertion and not to be eased through rest.

Form 6   Pull Toes with Both Hands

Starting Position: Stand at attention.

Movements:

A. Bend forward slowly, keeping legs straight, and hold toes with both hands. If you cannot reach them, just touch ankles with fingertips. Keep head a bit up (Fig. 7).

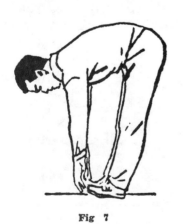

Fig 7

B. Return to starting position.

C. Place hands against the lower back and bend slowly backward.

D. Return to starting position.

Repeat these movements many times. Breathe as naturally as possible.

This is an exercise of the waist, which serves as the hinge for all body movements as well as a protector for some internal organs. It helps you not only to develop lumbar muscles and prevent and cure strains, but also to improve the functions of kidneys and adrenal.

But sufferers of hypertension and arteriosclerosis should not lower their head too much when doing this exercise.

Form 7   Clench Fists and Look with Eyes Wide Open

Starting Position: Take a ride-horse posture, toes gripping floor, hands tightly clenched beside waist, and knuckles turned down. Look ahead with eyes wide open (Fig. 8).

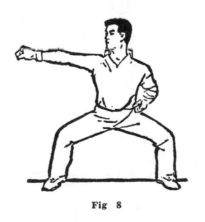

Fig 8

Movements:

A. Thrust right hand slowly rightward until arm is fully stretched, knuckles up.

B. Return to starting position.

C. Repeat A, reversing "right" to "left."

D. Return to starting position.

Repeat these movements many times. You may coordinate them with respiration, inhaling when you thrust fist and exhaling when you return to starting position.

This exercise helps to stimulate cerebral cortex and autonomic nerves, to promote blood circulation and to build up muscular strength and stamina.

Form 8   Rise and Fall On Tiptoes

Starting Position: Stand at attention, palms pressed against the front part of thighs and legs straightened.

Movements:

A. Raise both heels, drawing head up as if to lift a weight on its top.

B. Return to starting position.

Repeat these movements many times. You may coordinate them with respiration, inhaling when you raise heels and exhaling when you put them down.

This exercise causes light vibrations in the body to give finishing touches to the whole set of exercises.

Points to Remember

1. Exercise persistently. You'll never achieve the aim of keeping fit and preventing or

curing chronic diseases if you, as a Chinese saying goes, "go fishing for three days and dry the net for two."

2. When doing the exercises, relax yourself both physically and mentally. When exertion is needed, use force slowly and gently by "integrating hardness with softness" — a principle governing all traditional forms of fitness exercises in China.

3. Having achieved relaxation, think of the acupuncture point of dantian, 5 cm below the navel. Such thinking, which should not be too hard, will help abdominal respiration, promote blood circulation in the abdominal cavity and conduct qi to the lower part of your body.

4. Take a few deep breaths before you start the exercises. Breathe naturally and evenly. Practice in a place where the air is fresh.

5. Do not exercise within an hour after a meal.

6. The duration of a practice session and the intensity of exercise may vary from person to person. Generally speaking, it's enough when you start sweating lightly. In addition to baduanjin, you may take up some other fitness exercises which best suit your health condition, such as jogging, swimming, cold bath and sun bath.

YIJINJING

By ZHONG TI

Researcher, Beijing Qigong Society

Yijinjing literally means limbering-up exercise for the tendons. It is an ancient form of exercise in China, and is still used today by many people to keep themselves fit and improve their physique. It is not only good for health building but also serves as a kind of therapeutic exercise for orthopedic traumatic patients during their convalescence.

According to historical records, yijinjing was originally created and popularized as a means of strengthening the muscles and tendons. It is just as its name implies. "Yi" means limber up or strengthen. "Jin" means tendons and sinews. "Jing" means method.

The exercise is designed to turn flaccid and frail sinews and tendons into strong and sturdy ones. The movements of yijinjing are at once vigorous and gentle. Their performance calls for a unity of will and strength, i.e., using one's will to direct the exertion of muscular strength. It is coordinated with breathing.

The following is a brief introduction to the training methods.

There are 10 forms in this set of yijinjing. The starting position of each form requires that the eyes look straight ahead, the teeth are gritted tight together, the mouth is slightly open or closed but not tight, and the tongue rests on the hard palate.

Do not exert force, do not throw out the chest or raise the shoulders, and do not bend. Breathe naturally, keep relaxed, direct attention to the navel, and swallow the saliva when necessary. Be sure that each of these points is carried out throughout the exercise. These requirements will not be repeated when each of these forms is dealt with in detail below.

The main feature of this exercise is that all the movements are executed with the palms. At the beginning, each movement can be repeated eight or nine times. After a period of training, the number may be gradually increased to 30 times or more according to one's physical condition.

Form 1 Respiration with Fists Clenched

Starting Position: Stand with feet shoulder-width apart. Clench both fists with knuckles facing forward and tips of both thumbs pressed lightly against thighs (Fig. 1).

Method of Performing: Use gentle abdominal respiration. When breathing in, distend lower abdomen to the full. When breathing out, clench both fists tight. When inhaling again, continue to clench fists, and when exhaling, clench fists more tightly than before. Repeat these movements.

Form 2 Respiration with Palms Pressing Downward

Starting Position: Stand with feet shoulder-width apart. Press both palms downward with fingers pointing sideways and fingertips turned upward (Fig. 2).

Method of Performing: The method of breathing in and out

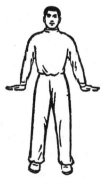

Fig 2

is the same as in Form 1. But when breathing out, press palms downward with inward strength. Do not bend legs. The whole body vibrates intensely.

When inhaling, keep body taut, and when exhaling again, press palms downward with more force and raise fingertips upward as much as possible, with body vibrating still more intensely. Repeat these movements.

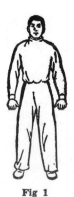

Fig 1

Form 3　Respiration with Palms Facing Upward

Starting Position: Stand with feet shoulder-width apart. Raise both arms shoulder-high sideways, with palms turned upward (Fig. 3).

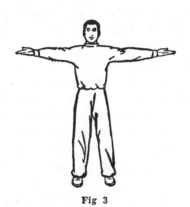

Fig 3

Method of Performing: Inhale to distend lower abdomen to the full. When breathing out, concentrate your mind on palms as if they were holding up heavy weights. Every time you breathe out, exert more inward strength as if the weight on palms were getting heavier and heavier. Keep the position of palms unchanged. Repeat these movements.

Form 4　Respiration with Palms Extending Outward

Starting Position: Stand with feet shoulder-width apart. Raise both arms shoulder-high sideways. The fingers point upward and palms face outward. Bend fingertips towards head as much as possible so that palms are extended outward (Fig. 4).

Method of Performing: Method of breathing is the same as before. When breathing out, extend palms outward with

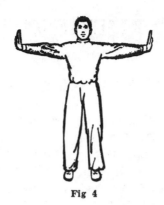

Fig 4

inward strength as if pushing something away, with the whole body vibrating intensely. Exert more force with each push so that you feel as if palms were extending further and further outward. Repeat these movements.

Form 5　Open and Close Respiration

Starting Position: Stand with feet shoulder-width apart. Place palms together in front of chest, with fingers turned upward and the tips of thumbs pressed against chest (Fig. 5a).

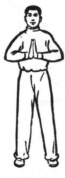

Fig 5a

Method of Performing: When breathing in, keep elbows level and draw palms slowly apart, with thumbs pressed lightly against chest, until they reach both sides of chest.
Meanwhile the whole body vibrates intensely (Fig. 5b). When breathing out, palms

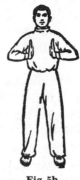

Fig 5b

move slowly towards each other to return to the starting position. The movements should coordinate with breathing, which should be slow, relaxed, gentle and even. Repeat these movements.

Form 6　Respiration with One Hand Propping Up And the Other Hanging Down

Starting Position: Move left foot a step to the left side to form a left "bow step," with left leg bent at knee and right leg fully stretched. Body is held straight naturally.
Raise left hand with palm facing upward, while right hand is hanging naturally by the right side of body, with fingertips pointing downward and palm facing thigh (Fig. 6a).

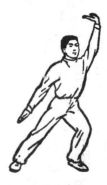

Fig 6a

Method of Performing: Throughout the breathing process, keep body position unchanged. While breathing, prop up left hand with inward strength, with right hand hanging down as if you were trying hard to extend arms as fully as possible.

Meanwhile the whole body vibrates intensely. Repeat these movements and relax naturally. Then move right foot a step to the right side to form a right bow step, and do the exercises in the reversed position (Fig. 6b).

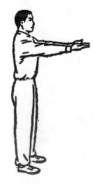

Fig 6b

Form 7   Rise and Fall Respiration

Starting Position: Stand with feet about 40 cm apart.

Method of Performing: Stretch both hands forward and raise them to shoulder level, with arms bent slightly and naturally and palms facing upward (Fig. 7a). Then turn

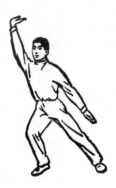

Fig 7a

palms downward (Fig. 7b), and at the same time squat down slowly while keeping trunk erect.

With the repetition of the movements, the squatting movement may progress gradually until thighs are parallel to the ground (Fig. 7c). Straighten up both legs slowly and turn both palms downward (Fig. 7d).

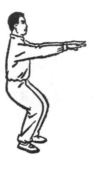

Fig 7b

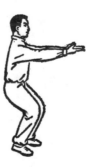

Fig 7c

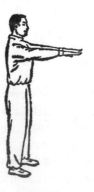

Fig 7d

In this form, inhale when raising hands and exhale when turning palms downward and squatting. Repeat the rise and fall breathing movements.

Persistent practice of this form not only will strengthen one's physique as a whole, but will help strengthen waist and do good to kidneys, thus enabling the trainee to walk with brisk steps.

Form 8   Respiration in Squatting Position

Starting Position: Stand with feet apart slightly more than shoulder-width apart. Put hands behind body with right fist clenched and left hand holding right wrist (Fig. 8).

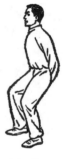

Fig 8

Method of Performing: Bend legs slightly and squat down a little. Maintain this position and do abdominal respiration. When breathing in, distend lower abdomen to the full. When breathing out, contract lower abdomen and elevate anus as if trying to hold back the stool. Repeat these movements.

This form is similar to the standing form in qigong. To a certain extent, it is useful in treating neurasthenia, hypertension and other ailments. Persistent practice will help strengthen lower limbs.

Form 9   Respiration in Bending Position

Starting Position: Stand with feet shoulder-width apart (Fig. 9a).

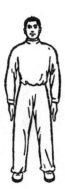

Fig 9a

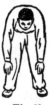

Fig 9b

Method of Performing: Bend body slowly to an angle of 90 degrees and at the same time let the hands hang down naturally (Fig. 9b).

Shoulders should vibrate slightly as hands drop slowly, with palms turned inward and fingertips pointing downward. Do not exert any strength with hands. Inhale when bending forward and exhale when straightening up. Repeat these movements.

This form will help reduce excess fat in abdomen and cure lumbago and backache.

Form 10   Respiration While Twisting Body

Starting Position: Stand at attention.

Method of Performing: Move left foot a step to the left side to form a left bow step. Twist body to the left, with left hand placed on the back part of waist and palm facing outward. Bend right arm to form an arch and place it over forehead, with palm facing outward and about a fist's distance away from forehead. Keep eyes on right heel which remains on the ground (Fig. 10a).

As body twists to the left while forming a left bow step, waist is in a tense condition. When breathing out, imagine that the center of gravity is shifted to right heel. Gradually increase the degree of waist turning, and try to breathe with the help of abdomen (Fig. 10a).

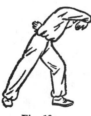

Fig 10a

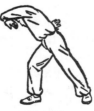

Fig 10b

Repeat the above movements, reversing "right" and "left" (Fig. 10b).

Persistent practice of this form will help prevent and cure lumbago and backache.

TAIJI QIGONG

By JI TI

Researcher, National Research Institute of Sports Science

Taiji qigong is a simple and effective exercise popular in China. If done persistently, it helps the weak to get stronger and the healthy to grow more energetic and live a longer life. It has special curative effects on certain chronic diseases, such as troubles of the digestive, respiratory and nervous systems, as well as heart disease, hypertension, rheumatism, and arthritis.

Taiji qigong is easy to learn, consisting as it does of just a few movements. By following carefully the methods of training and points for attention, one can do the exercise without the help of a teacher. Following are four ways of practicing it and points for attention.

I.   Standing Form

Starting Position: Stand with toes of both feet turned inward (in reversed splayfeet position), big toes being one-sixth of a meter apart and heels one-third of a meter apart. The weight of body mainly rests on balls of feet.

Keep both knees straight and upright, shoulders expanded and chest out. Lower abdomen is drawn in and head slightly inclined forward.

The center of gravity is on both feet. Concentrate the mind on dantian, the acupuncture point about 5 cm below the navel. Close eyes slightly, look at the tip of nose and listen to the breathing.

Movement 1. Stand in the same starting position as before, with hands hanging down naturally against sides of both legs. Take deep breaths abdominally, inhaling through nose and exhaling through mouth.

Breathing should be slow, deep and even. Raise the tip of tongue against hard palate while inhaling, and return it to normal position while exhaling.

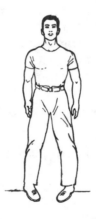

Movement 1

The breaths should go deep down to the lower abdomen. An inhaling and exhaling makes one breath. Silently count 15 breaths before proceeding to the second movement.

Movement 2. Extend both arms straight ahead at shoulder level, palms facing outward and fingers point upward.

Points for attention:

A. The thumb and fingers of both hands should be held close together.

B. Keep mouth closed and raise the tip of tongue against hard palate.

C. Breathe in and out naturally through nose. Breathing should be slow and even. Silently count 10 breaths before proceeding to the third movement.

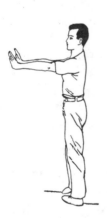

Movement 2

Movement 3. Stand in the same starting position as before. Stretch both arms sideways at shoulder level to form a straight line. The palms face sideward and fingers point upward. The points for attention are the same as in movement 2. Also, count 10 breaths before proceeding to the fourth movement.

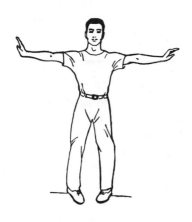

Movement 3

Movement 4. Stand in the same starting position as before. Extend both arms backward, palms facing downward and fingers held close together.

Press arms tightly against ribs, with chest inclined forward at about 30 degrees. Raise both arms as high as possible without moving body.

The points for attention are the same as in the second movement. Count 15 breaths.

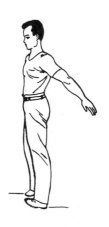

Movement 4

The above four movements should be performed continuously. The reversed

splayfeet position is the basic form which remains unchanged throughout the four movements. Move arms and hands only. Take 50 breaths altogether to complete the series of movements.

After every two weeks, add three breaths to movement 1, two to movement 2, two to movement 3 and three to movement 4, adding up to an increase of 10 breaths in all. Thus, after two and a half months, the number of breaths in the four movements will be 100.

Carry on in this way for three months before further increasing the number of breaths in accordance with one's health and the time available. But in all cases the increase should be gradual.

II.   Sitting Form

Sit on bed. Stretch legs straight, and keep toes of both feet together and heels apart to form the reversed splayfeet stance. Hold the stretched fingers close together, with knuckles facing upward, and tuck hands under thighs. Hold chest out and draw in lower abdomen. The head inclines slightly forward.

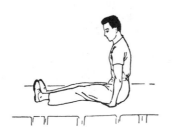

Sitting Form

Concentrate the mind on the acupoint of dantian about 5 cm below navel. Keep mouth closed

and raise the tip of tongue against hard palate. Close eyes slightly, look at the tip of nose and listen to the breathing.

Breathe naturally in and out of nose, with the breaths going deep down to lower abdomen. Silently count 100 breaths (or 50 if one is weak after illness).

Add 10 breaths after every two weeks, so that the number of breaths is increased gradually from 110 to 150, 160, and 200, depending on the condition of your health. Be careful not to catch cold in cold weather.

III.   Lying Form

Lie on back in bed. Stretch legs straight, and keep big toes about one-third of a meter apart and heels a little wider apart to form a reversed splayfeet stance. Hold the stretched fingers close together, with knuckles facing upward, and put hands under thighs. Rest head on a pillow, with shoulders in a naturally relaxed position.

Other movements are the same as in the sitting form. Silently count 100 breaths (50 at the beginning if one is weak after illness). Follow the same rate of increase as in the sitting form.

As one can usually practice longer while lying on one's back, the number of breaths can be increased to 300. Further increases will have to depend on the condition of one's health. In cold weather, cover the body with a blanket so as not to catch cold.

IV.   Walking Form

Put both hands behind the back, left hand forming a hollow fist and held in palm of right hand. Forearms are pressed gently against upper part of buttocks. Relax shoulders and chest, and incline head slightly forward. Walk slowly and in a relaxed manner. The eyes and attention concentrate on toes and the ears listen to the breathing. Breathing should coordinate with the steps.

The principle is to take several steps for each inhalation and the same number of steps for each exhalation. The length of inhalation and exhalation should be even. The number of steps taken should be increased gradually — from two steps for each inhalation and exhalation to nine steps.

Take deep breaths abdominally, inhaling through nose and exhaling through mouth. It is advisable to do this exercise in the fields or woods where the air is fresh. Do it as if you are taking a stroll, and never mind about the time and distance.

V.   Five Essential Points

In order to obtain the desired results, the following five points should be observed:

1. The mind should rest at ease and remain tranquil.
2. The posture and movements should be correct.
3. Breathe slowly.
4. Increase the length of time for the exercise gradually.
5. Keep on doing the exercise regularly every day.

VI.   Points of Attention

1. The standing form is the essential part of the exercise. The walking form can be done as a means of relaxing the body, after going through the movements in the sitting or lying position.
2. Do the exercise in a quiet place where the air is fresh, preferably where trees, flowers and other plants are grown.
3. It is preferable to do the standing exercise once after getting up in the morning and once before going to bed and do the sitting exercise before taking a noon nap. The walking exercise should be done after the standing exercise. If there is not enough time, at least do the standing exercise once after getting up in the morning, or do the sitting or lying exercise before getting up.
4. In rainy, foggy or windy weather, do the exercise indoors.
5. Stop doing the exercise for some time if you have a cold or fever or if you vomit blood.
6. Don't do the standing exercise within half an hour after a meal. The sitting or lying exercise, however, can be done after a little rest. The walking exercise can be done at any time.
7. Do not drink cold water immediately after the exercise. Take care not to catch cold if you should sweat.
8. Wear loose clothes when you do the exercise.
9. Do not talk with others when you do the exercise. If anyone should interrupt you, start all over again.
10. Women who are three months pregnant should stop doing the exercise.

VII.   At the beginning one may experience these reactions:

1. Limbs ache.
2. Palms turn cold.
3. Arms shiver.
4. Chest and knees feel distended.

Don't worry if you have these reactions, because they are quite normal. Keep on doing the exercise and they will disappear in a few days. After some time, however, one may have other reactions such as breaking wind, hiccuping, perspiring, or having a fever. These are good symptoms. In three or four months, there will be more saliva in your mouth when you do the exercise and you will feel a slightly sweet taste. In six months, you will feel extremely comfortable every time after doing the exercise. But if you stop doing it, you will feel rather uncomfortable.

WUQIN QIGONG

By LI GAOZHONG

Reporter, Sports News

In Sichuan, which is known as the land of abundance in southwest China, people in the tens of thousands practice "wuqin qigong" every morning or evening in the parks, playgrounds and qigong coaching centers.

Wuqin qigong is a kind of internal breathing exercise in wushu, with a history of about 2,000 years. It is very popular among the people in Sichuan and is effective in preventing and curing diseases.

Wuqinxi, meaning five-animal play, was devised by the well-known physician Hua Tuo (?-203) over 1,000 years earlier than a kind of therapeutical exercise evolved by a Swede. It was passed on to Hua's disciple Wu Pu and then handed down from generation to generation. It was said that Yue Fei (1103-1142), a famous general of the Song Dynasty (960-1279), often practiced this exercise. As it spread among the people, many schools were evolved, one of which was wuqin qigong.

Animal Movements Mimicked

Wuqin qigong mimics the movements, features and postures of apes, deer, tigers, bears, and birds, accompanied by breathing exercise. The aim is to enhance the functions of the internal organs, nerves, muscles and bones as well as to prevent and cure diseases, and to improve one's health and prolong one's life.

The "ape" form of qigong (Photo 1) is the basic exercise for the weak to become strong. It mainly exercises the lower abdomen and helps improve the functions of the kidneys. The "deer" form (Photo 2) is good for the upper abdomen and has the effect of strengthening the stomach and the spleen. The "tiger" form (Photo 3) is designed especially for the chest and the back. After training for a long period of time, one can develop a sonorous voice, renewed vigour and nimbleness in action.

For the waist, the "bear" form (Photo 4) has special effects. The functions of the liver and kidneys, too, will be greatly improved. Doing the "bird" form (Photo 5) is salubrious to the heart and the spine. It is also good for the nerves and helps keep the blood pressure normal.

In addition, there are two kinds of exercises of a higher standard. One is called the "head" form (Photo 6), which helps to strengthen the brains, and the other is called the "bottom" form which is good for the testicles. The latter form is similar to the former in posture, the only difference being that the toes touch the ground.

One difference between wuqin qigong and other types of qigong lies in "paiqi," or "beating." As shown in Photo 7, this method consists in using an outside force (a pouch of iron sand or a little hammer) to beat the relevant "jingluo" and acupuncture points so as to produce an impact on the diseased part of the body and help the transmission of qi and circulation of blood in the body.

In traditional Chinese medicine, "jingluo" refers to the main and collateral channels in the human body, regarded as a network of passages through which vital energy circulates and along which the acupuncture points are distributed. These are sometimes called acupuncture meridians. The beating has the efficacy of treating chronic diseases and lumps in the body which cannot be cured with ordinary medicines or by massaging.

Large numbers of people in Sichuan learn and practice wuqin qigong, because the exercises are simple and easy to grasp and suitable for various age groups of both sexes, and produce no side effects. Many patients suffering from chronic diseases or cancer have obtained good results after a period of serious exercise.

Many Improvements Reported

Huang Ruxin, a 60-year-old retired worker of the Chongqing Cement Plant, suffered from cancer of the throat and gave up all hope of being cured since the malignant growth was in a late stage. He did not even bother to have an operation, for the doctor had pronounced it to be incurable. But to the doctor's astonishment, his health and his voice gradually recovered after he had taken up the wuqin qigong exercises for one year. That was six years ago, and today he is still going strong.

Another example is Cao Yanzeng, a woman patient who had been bed-ridden for more than one year because of osteomyelitis. When she started learning qigong, she had to hobble to a coaching center with the help of others. But now she can walk by herself and her health has greatly improved.

There are many other examples — people suffering from cirrhosis, pulmonary emphysema, coronary heart disease, hypertension, neurosis and so forth. They all say that wuqin qigong helps cure diseases and keeps one healthy and fit.

Now, a scientific research center for qigong has been set up in the city of Chongqing, using modern scientific methods to study the therapeutical effects of wuqin qigong.

In one of the qigong coaching centers in Chongqing, this writer interviewed Yu Dehua and Xiang Yanghui, both qigong masters and compilers of the book "Wuqin Qigong." Ye Dehua, 73, is a retired worker of the Chongqing Cement Plant. When he was 18, he was very weak and was plagued with illnesses. He began to learn wuqin qigong from local qigong masters, with the result that he was cured of hernia and other diseases and he could walk scores of kilometers a day without effort. For more than 50 years he has persisted in practicing wuqin qigong, and today he is as vigorous as a young man.

Xiang Yanhui is an old editor of the Chongqing Daily. On the basis of traditional Chinese medicine, he and Yu Dehua cooperated in compiling and collating the book "Wuqin Qigong," which is very popular among the people. Apart from teaching qigong in Chongqing, they answer letters from various parts of the country and abroad.

Now wuqin qigong is not only practiced in Sichuan, but has spread to many other provinces in China.

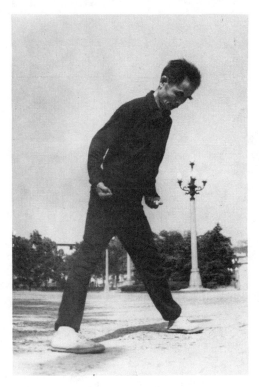

Photo 1: The ape form.

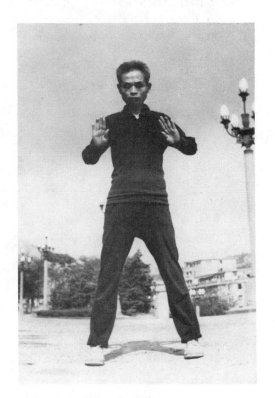

Photo 2: The deer form.

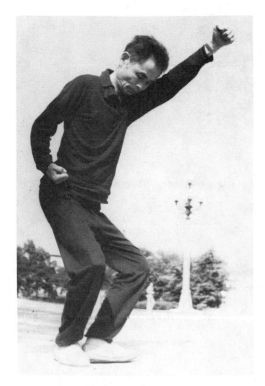

Photo 3: The tiger form.

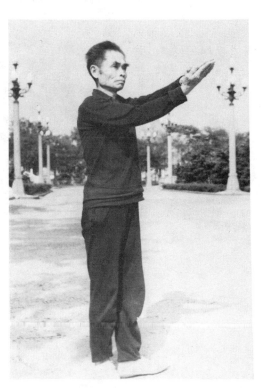

Photo 4: the bear form.

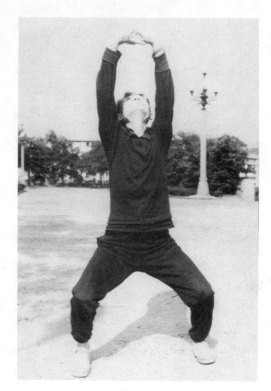

Photo 5: The bird form.

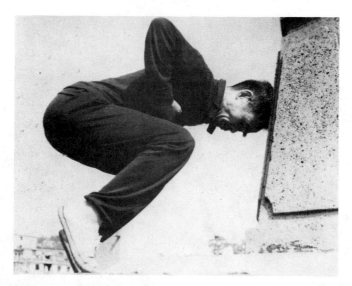

Photo 6: The head form.

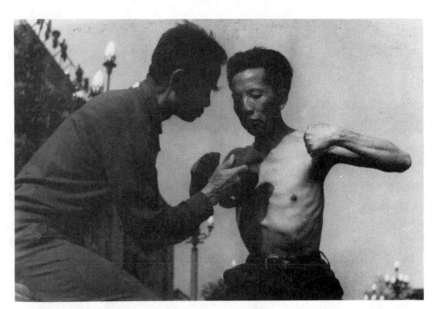

Photo 7: Yu Dehua (left) performs beating exercise on Huan Ruxin, who is under treatment for cancer.

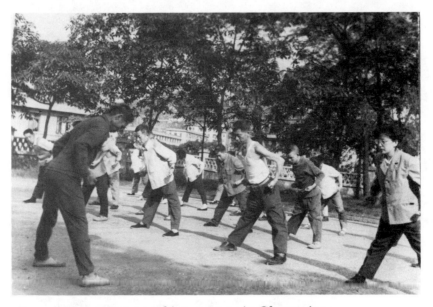

One of the qigong coaching centers in Chongqing.

PHOTOS BY: Li Gaozhong

DAYAN QIGONG: WILD GOOSE BREATHING EXERCISE

(First 64 Forms)

By YANG MEIJUN

A well-known woman qigong master in Beijing

I.   A Brief Introduction

Dayan Qigong, literally meaning Wild Goose Breathing Exercise, is a set of highly salubrious exercises handed down through the ages among exclusive circles of the Taoist Kunlun School. Imitating the postures and movements of the wild goose and assimilating the ancient daoyin methods, it consists of both vigorous and gentle movements in which motion is alternated with stillness. By stimulating a strong sensation of qi, it provides an effective cure for diseases.

The first 64 forms of the exercise as described in the following pages, take only 5-10 minutes to complete, and are particularly suitable for mental workers of middle or old age. The movements, though rather numerous, are easy to learn, and may be practiced either as a whole or part by part.

Dayan Qigong helps promote blood circulation and clear jingmai, or the passages through which vital energy flows. It helps the performer to take in health-giving air from nature and to discharge foul air from his body. It also enables him to quickly master the art of emitting waiqi (outflowing air) to cure diseases for himself or for other people. It is particularly good for such ailments as hypertension and hypotension, heart diseases, neurasthenia, insomnia, functional disorder of autonomic nerves, gastrointestinal problems, rheumatoid arthritis and skin diseases. It also helps to take off fat from the obese.

For the middle-aged and older people, it serves as a kind of therapy for self-regulation and self-repair, one that benefits the human body as an organic whole. Unlike medical treatment, it has no side effects. An old man who practices the exercise for two or three months will find his muscles much more supple, his joints in the waist, legs, shoulders and arms more flexible, his cerebral functions improved and his memory strengthened. In a word, Dayan Qigong helps to delay aging and prolong life.

II.   Methods of Exercise

1. baihui 2. yintang 3. right quepen
4. right qihu 5. shenque (navel)
6. hegu 7. tanzhong 8. left quepen
9. left qihu 10. left shenyu
11. right shenyu 12. baihui 13. taiyang

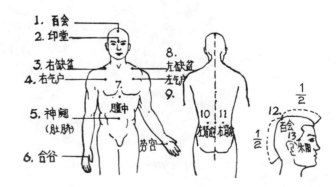

Acupuncture Points

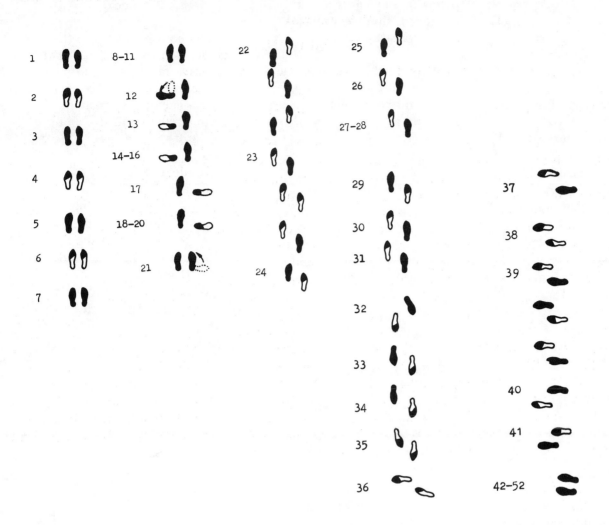

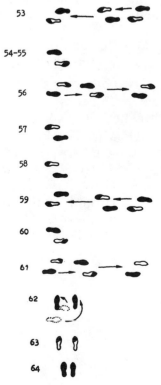

Footwork Patterns

Form 1   Starting Position

Stand erect with feet parallel and shoulder-width apart. Imagine you are propping up something with your head. Keep shoulders relaxed and arms hanging naturally at your sides, with palms turned inward, fingers naturally separated and slightly flexed. Close your mouth slightly and rest your tongue lightly on the hard palate. Look straight ahead (Fig. 1).

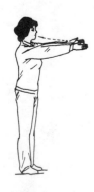

Fig 1

Relax your whole body and remain calm and quiet. Keep your qi down to the lower abdomen. Rid your mind of all distracting thoughts and stand quietly for a while.

Form 2   Spread Wings

Raise both arms slowly to the front, with palms facing each other, until they come shoulder high (Fig. 2). Then, as you go on raising arms, spread them

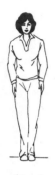

Fig 2

out and rotate them so that palms face upwards, chest expanded, shoulders relaxed and elbows slightly bent.

Meanwhile, bend body backward and lift heels slightly off floor with knees slightly flexed. Look up to the sky (Fig. 3).

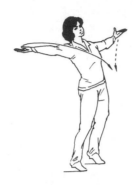

Fig 3

Points for attention: When you bend your body backward and look up to the sky, see that you do not overdo it lest you lose your balance or feel bad.

Form 3   Close Wings

Rotate arms inward and bring hands down to the front of abdomen with arms rounded, palms turned inward. Fingers of both hands point at each other, about 10 cm apart, thumb and forefinger forming a curve.

As you bring your hands down to the front, restore body to erect position, draw in abdomen and set heels down on floor. Look down to the front (Fig. 4).

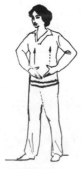

Fig 4

Form 4   Draw Wings to The Back

Lift both hands up to the chest, palms still facing inward. Rotate arms inward and turn palms so that they face each other. Then consciously put forth strength and stretch arms forward while lifting heels off floor.

Rotate arms inward so as to turn hands back to back (Fig. 5). Spread out arms vigorously and swing them down to the back of the hips with palms turned backward. Look straight ahead.

Relax shoulders and keep armpits "empty" (with enough space to hold an egg under each arm). Heels are still off floor (Fig. 6).

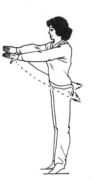

Fig 5

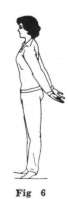

Fig 6

Form 5   Jerk Arms

Bend elbows and lift hands up to your back with palms

turning up and fingers curling back in the form of a claw (Fig. 7).

Rotating arms outward, bring your clawed hands up on your back and then suddenly out into the front for a backhand punch, elbows bent at 90 degrees. Fingers point to the front and palms face upward and a bit inward.

At the same time as you execute the backhand punch, quickly snap your upper arms against your sides and bring your heels down on floor. Look straight ahead (Fig. 8).

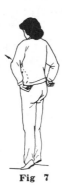

Fig 7

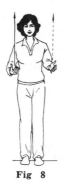

Fig 8

Form 6 Draw Wings to The Back

Rotate arms inward as they extend forward with palms facing each other. Meanwhile, lift heels off floor and continue to rotate arms inward until hands are back to back. Then repeat movements as shown in Figs. 5-6.

Form 7 Jerk Arms

Same as Form 5.

Form 8 Lift Arms

Slowly lift arms with palms facing inward and fingers pointing up, until hands come above head level. Elbows are bent in front with shoulders relaxed. Look straight ahead (Fig. 9).

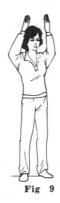

Fig 9

Form 9 Clasp Hands

Rotating arms inward, clasp hands overhead with fingers interlaced, palms facing the acupuncture point *baihui* at top of head (Fig. 10).

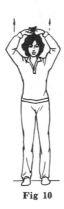

Fig 10

Form 10 Turn up Palms

Rotate arms inward so that palms are turned up. Then apply strength consciously to stretch arms upward. Look upward to the front. Legs are straightened while feet stay still (Fig. 11).

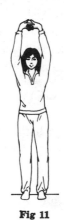

Fig 11

Form 11 Bend Waist (Forward, Left and Right)

Bend body forward with legs straightened. Clasp hands with fingers straight and interlaced. Press them toward the floor with palm side down. Keep them between the feet for a while (Fig. 12).

Then lift torso up a bit and turn to the left before pressing clasped hands down to the front of left foot. Keep them there for a while, then lift them up a bit and turn torso to the right before pressing clasped hands down to the front of right foot. Keep them there for a while. Eyes follow hands. Top of head points downward or forward. Position of feet is unchanged throughout.

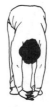

Fig 12

Points for attention: Try your best to touch the floor with your clasped hands. The beginner, however, should not over-exert himself. The old and the sick are not required to bend too low, but in any circumstances one must keep one's legs straightened.

Form 12 Twine Hands

Lift hands a little off floor and turn torso so that it faces square to the front. Separate hands to both sides with fingers pointing at each other and palms turned down. Turn left foot 90 degrees to the left.

Meanwhile, with knees slightly flexed and using waist as pivot, lift torso up a bit and turn it 90 degrees to the left while swinging arms in harmony with the waist turn. The right arm rotates inward (palm turned out) and swings out to the front and then to the left (Fig. 13).

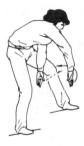

Fig 13

Then rotate both arms outward so as to turn palms up and cross forearms in front of abdomen, right arm on top (Fig. 14).

When you rotate arms and turn palms up, twist right hip and right leg quickly to the right and swing right arm towards right hip, with right leg bent and left leg straightened, left foot flat on floor. Eyes follow right hand.

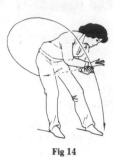

Fig 14

Form 13 Recover Air

Bring fingers of left hand together to form a claw and lift them up to the acupoint *quepen* (on left collarbone) while relaxing left shoulder and leaving left armpit empty. Right hand continues to swing down to the right.

When right arm is straightened, swing it up at the back and then down to the front in a giant circle until right hand comes down on left toes.

In harmony with the arm swing, turn torso to the left and bend it forward in that direction. Your feet are now in a "T" stance, with right leg bent at knee while left leg is straightened, left heel on floor and left toes turned up. Weight rests on right foot. Look at right hand (Fig. 15).

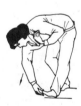

Fig 15

Form 14 Pull Left Toes (three times)

Grip the first two toes of left foot with right hand and pull them back three times while slightly bending right arm and thrusting right elbow outward.

In coordination with the movement of right hand, turn shoulder, waist and hips to the left three times. Look at right hand. Feet position remains unchanged.

Points for attention: Apply as much strength as will make you comfortable. Relax shoulders, waist and hips. Instead of gripping the toes, the old and the sick may just point their right hand towards the left foot, but they are still required to turn the waist and thrust the elbow outward three times.

Form 15 Push Air

Letting go of the toes, open right hand and separate fingers, with thumb and forefinger forming a curve and palm turning backward to the right.

Bending right arm slightly, exert strength consciously to push right hand slowly backward to the right while torso turns slowly in the same direction (for about 45 degrees), with waist and hips relaxed.

Eyes follow right hand. Weight rests on right foot. Feet position remains unchanged (Fig. 16).

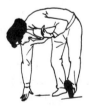

Fig 16

Form 16 Scoop Up Air

As right arm is pushed to the back of right hip, rotate it outward so that palm faces front left, fingers pointing downward. With right arm slightly bent, exert strength consciously to "scoop up air" — moving the hand up to front left while wrist is gradually flexed, palm turned up.

Fingers point in the direction of the scooping movement. Coordinate torso turn with movement of right hand. Eyes follow right hand. Feet position remain unchanged (Fig. 17).

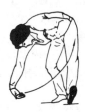

Fig 17

Form 17 Turn Body and Recover Air

When right hand comes to the front of chest, close fingers to form a claw with tips pointing up and resting on right collarbone. Meanwhile, using right heel as pivot, turn body 180 degrees to the right and shift weight onto left foot.

Bend left knee and drop left hand before swinging left arm forward, upward, backward, downward, and forward again in a giant circle that ends with left hand falling on the toes of right foot.

Eyes follow left hand. Toes of right foot are turned up. Right heel rests on floor (Fig. 18).

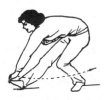

Fig 18

Form 18 Pull Right Toes

Same as Form 14 except that "right" and "left" are reversed.

Form 19 Push Air

Same as Form 15 except that "right" and "left" are reversed.

Form 20 Scoop Up Air

Same as Form 16 except that "right" and "left" are reversed.

Form 21 Twine Hands

Bring left hand up to abdomen in a scooping movement. Meanwhile, open right hand with thumb and forefinger forming a curve. Lower it to the inner side of left hand as you straighten up body and turn to the left, right foot turning 90 degrees to the left so that it is parallel to left foot again.

Then right hand moves downward, outward, upward and backward while left hand moves outward, upward, backward, and downward so that the two hands circle around each other three times with palms facing inward, about 16 cm apart.

In coordination with the hand movements, sway your waist, hips and shoulders naturally from side to side (Fig. 19).

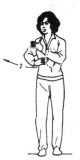

Fig 19

Form 22 Wave Hands Like Clouds

1. Wave Right Hand

Withdraw left hand to left hip with arm bent and palm turned upward and slightly inward. Right hand extends to the front at waist level with palm turned up. Meanwhile, bring right foot half a step forward with external side of ball of foot on floor. Weight rests on left foot. Look at right palm (Fig. 20).

Move right arm rightward and to the back in a curve while torso twists in the same direction. Eyes follow right hand. Then rotate right arm inward and bend arm with palm turned up so that *hegu* acupuncture point on right hand is pressed against right *shenyu* point on lumber vertebra.

Meanwhile, turn torso to the left so that it faces square to the front while lifting left heel off floor and transferring weight onto right foot. Look straight ahead.

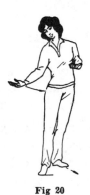

Fig 20

2. Wave Left Hand

While shifting weight onto right foot with *hegu* point on right hand pressed against right *shenyu* point, move left foot

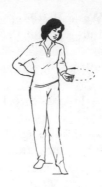

Fig 21

half a step forward with external side of ball of foot on floor (Fig. 21).

Meanwhile, reach out right hand and then draw it leftward and to the back in a horizontal curve while twisting torso to the left in coordination with hand movement.

Then rotate left arm inward and bend elbow so that *hegu* point on left hand is pressed against left *shenyu* point on lumbar vertebra.

Meanwhile, turn torso back to normal position, shift weight onto left foot and lift right heel off floor. Look straight ahead.

3. Wave Right Hand

Same as in the previous section (Fig. 20).

Form 23 Twist Waist

Move left foot half a step forward with ball of foot on floor. Meanwhile, extend left hand out to the front (Fig. 22).

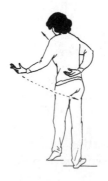

Fig 22

Then move left hand in a curve to the back of left hip, while twisting torso to the left and carrying right arm up to front left with elbow flexed and upper arm brought up to shoulder level, hand hanging naturally with palm facing inward and fingers pointing downward.

Body leans forward to the left, weight rests on left foot, and both heels are lifted off floor. Look at left hand (Fig. 23). Then twist torso

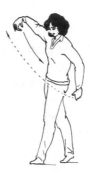

Fig 23

quickly to the right and swing both arms in coordination — right arm rotating outward and swinging back to right hip with elbow bent at about 90 degrees, palm turned up and fingers pointing forward.

Left arm "scoops" up to the front until palm faces *yintang* point. Elbow is flexed so that upper arm and forearm form a curve.

Meanwhile, torso, waist and hips are all restored to normal

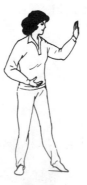

Fig 24

position. Right heel lands quickly on floor and left heel is lifted off floor. Weight is shifted onto right foot. Both knees are slightly bent. Look at left palm (Fig. 24).

Form 24 Drop Arm to Recover Air

Rotate left arm inward so as to turn palm downward (Fig. 25). Bring left hand down to the side of left buttock with palm facing backward and fingers pointing downward. Look straight ahead (Fig. 26).

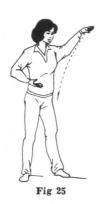

Fig 25

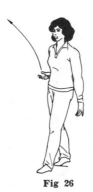

Fig 26

Form 25 Spread Single Wing

Shift weight onto left foot and move right foot half a step forward with ball of foot on floor. Carry right hand upward and forward to shoulder level with palm turned up, fingers apart, thumb and forefinger forming a curve.

Then move right arm to the right in a horizontal curve while turning torso in the same direction. Eyes follow right palm (Fig. 27).

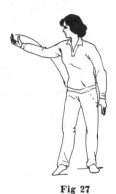

Fig 27

When right arm has moved backward to the right, rotate it inward and bend elbow before bringing it down to the right and the back in a curve until *hegu* point is pressed against right *shenyu* point, palm turned up.

Meanwhile, restore torso to normal position and shift weight onto right foot. Look straight ahead.

Form 26 Step Forward and Extend Arm

Move left foot half a step forward with external side of ball of foot on floor. Meanwhile, rotate left arm outward and lift it up until elbow is bent about 90 degrees at waist side. The palm is turned upward and slightly inward. Fingers point forward. Look at left palm (Fig. 28).

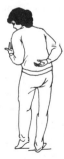

Fig 28

Form 27 Wind Hand Around Head and Ears

With feet position unchanged, turn torso to the left with waist as pivot while lowering right hand and turning palm inward before bringing it up to the front of abdomen.

Along with the leftward body turn, bring the right hand further up to the left side. Then right hand winds past left shoulder, left ear and nape until right palm is turned towards left ear and neck (Fig. 29).

When right hand passes nape, turn torso and head square to the front. Then go on moving right hand around the neck until palm faces right ear, with shoulder relaxed and elbow bent and pointing to front right. Look straight ahead (Fig. 30).

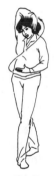

Fig 29

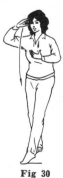

Fig 30

Form 28 Press Downward

Exert strength consciously to press right hand down to the side of right hip, palm facing downward, wrist flexed back, fingers pointing forward and separated. Thumb and forefinger form a curve.

Meanwhile, lift left hand up to shoulder level until elbow is slightly bent, palm turned upward and slightly inward. Look at left hand. Feet position unchanged. Weight still on right foot (Fig. 31).

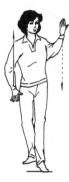

Fig 31

Form 29 Prop Up

Rotate right arm outward and turn up palm as you bring right hand forward and upward in a curve to shoulder level. Palm faces upward and slightly inward, elbow slightly bent.

Meanwhile, lower left hand to left side. Look at right palm. Shift weight onto left foot and lift right heel off floor (Fig. 32).

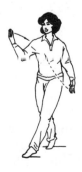

Fig 32

Form 30 Recover Air

Rotate right arm inward quickly and bend elbow. With elbow pointing to the right, close fingers to form a claw and place it on the right *quepen* point. Meanwhile, carry left hand in a scooping movement up to the front with palm facing inward and fingers pointing up. *Laogong* point on the palm faces *yintang* point on the head. Look at left palm.

In coordination with arm movements, quickly shift weight onto right foot with knee slightly bent and lift left heel off floor (Fig. 33).

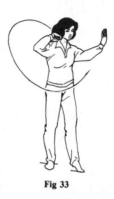

Fig 33

Form 31 Scoop the Moon

Bend right leg as weight rests on right foot, and straighten left leg naturally with external side of ball of foot on floor. Keep left arm where it is. Open fingers of right hand so that thumb and forefinger form a curve.

Then carry right arm backward to the right in a smooth movement while torso turns in the same direction. Eyes follow right hand. Then rotate right arm outward and drop it down before moving it up to the left in a curve while torso twists in the same direction and leans forward.

When moving up in a curve, right arm should pass over

lower abdomen before going up to the external side of left forearm to form a cross with it while both palms turn inward. Look at right palm (Fig. 34).

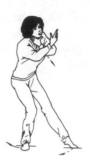

Fig 34

Form 32 Turn Body

Using both feet as pivot, slowly turn 180 degrees to the right. Bend left leg and shift weight onto left foot while right heel is lifted slightly off floor and buttocks are drawn in. Keep torso erect.

In coordination with body turn, lower left hand past chest and abdomen and down to the left side with palm turned backward and fingers pointing downward and to the back.

Meanwhile, slowly raise right arm and bend elbow with palm facing inward and fingers pointing upward, *laogong* point facing *yintang* point. Look at right palm (Fig. 35).

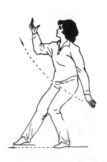

Fig 35

Form 33 Step Forward and Look at Palm

Shift weight onto right foot and bring left foot one step forward with ball of foot on floor.

Meanwhile, rotate left arm outward and lift it up to the front with elbow bent and palm turned inward, fingers pointing up and *laogong* point facing *yintang* point. Look at left palm.

While moving left arm, carry right hand slightly to the right so that palm faces right temple (Fig. 36).

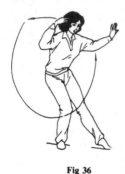

Fig 36

Form 34 Look up to The Moon

Lift internal side of ball of left foot slightly off floor and squat deeply on right leg. Keeping left hand where it is, extend right arm to the right while torso twists towards the same direction.

Then rotate right arm outward and bring it downward to the left in a curve while torso twists towards the left.

As torso leans forward to the left, right hand curves under left arm and then snaps up with palm turned upward and fingers pointing to upper left. Meanwhile, turn your head to the left and look up at the sky (Fig. 37).

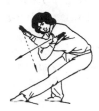

Fig 37

Form 35 Press Air

Rotate both arms inward so that palms are turned down, fingers separated, thumb and forefinger forming a curve, while torso is turned square to the front and lifted up to erect position.

Then bend both knees with left knee in front and with right foot and right knee turned slightly inward, both heels off floor, weight on right foot.

Meanwhile, place hands on either side of left knee with fingers pointing at each other. When squatting down, exert strength consciously to press palms downward with wrists flexed back.

Then rise up a little and at the same time bring hands up with wrists and fingers naturally relaxed. In this way, squat down and rise up three times. Look at hands (Fig. 38).

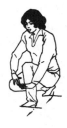

Fig 38

Form 36 Turn Body and Press Air

Keep hands where they are. Using balls of feet as pivot, turn 90 degrees to the right so that right foot is in front and left foot and left knee are turned inward, heels off floor. Then do the squat-and-rise movements as in Form 35 (Fig. 39).

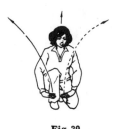

Fig 39

Form 37 Swim Forward

Rise up and straighten legs with weight on right foot and left heel lifted off floor. Meanwhile, straighten arms naturally with wrists relaxed and fingers pointing forward.

Then, with hands and arms quivering, lift arms forward with palms facing down, then upward to both sides with palms turned forward. Look straight ahead.

Meanwhile, shift weight backward and set left heel on floor while lifting right heel off floor (Fig. 40).

Keep hands and arms quivering all the time until Form 42.

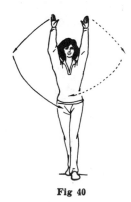

Fig 40

Form 38 Look Down at Water

Shift weight onto right foot and lift left heel off floor.

Meanwhile, rotate arms inward and quiver them while spreading them apart and then lowering them to the back in a curve with palms facing each other, body slightly leaning forward, heels (or only left heel) off floor. Look down to the front (Fig. 41).

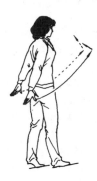

Fig 41

Then, with arms still quivering, slowly raise them forward and upward to shoulder level with palm facing downward and fingers pointing forward.

Meanwhile, shift weight backward onto left foot and lift right heel slightly off floor while body leans slightly backward. Look straight ahead.

Form 39 Pat Water and Fly Away

1. Pat Water on Left

With weight on left foot, move quivering arms slowly in a curve forward and upward to the left while torso twists leftward and bends slightly forward.

Left hand is brought higher than head level with palm facing outward and thumb pointing down, while right hand comes to chest level with palm facing downward and slightly to the left. Both arms are slightly

bent. Look at left hand
(Fig. 42).

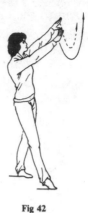

Fig 42

2. Pat Water on Right

Shift weight forward onto
right foot and lift left heel
off floor while moving the
quivering arms to the front with
torso turning back to normal
position. Look straight ahead.

Then move quivering arm
slowly in a curve to the right
while torso twists towards the
same direction and bends
slightly forward.

Right hand is brought higher
than head level with palm
facing outward and thumb
pointing down, while left hand
comes to chest level with palm
facing downward and slightly to
the right. Look at right hand
(Fig. 43).

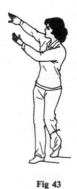

Fig 43

3. Pat Water on Left

Same as in Fig. 42.

All the movements in this
form must be continuous with
arms quivering all the time.

Form 40 Drink Water
(three times)

Shift weight onto right foot
and lift heel off floor. With
arms still shaking, move them
to the front at shoulder level
while turning torso back to
normal position. Look straight
ahead.

Now move left foot a step
forward and place ball of foot
on floor while separating the
quivering arms and bringing
hands down to the sides with
palms facing downward.

Then bend right knee deeply
and straighten left leg naturally
while bending torso forward.
Meanwhile, bend elbows and
withdraw hands to hips before
reaching them down and out to
the front of left foot, palms still
facing downward and fingers
pointing forward, head lifted up
and eyes looking down to the
front.

The movement is reminiscent
of a wild goose drinking water
by the side of a stream
(Fig. 44).

Then lift up torso and draw
hands up to hips with elbows
bent. Do the "drink-water"
movement three times.

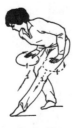

Fig 44

Form 41 Gaze at the Sky

Slowly draw up arms
(Fig. 45) and straighten up body

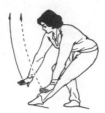

Fig 45

while shifting weight forward
onto left foot and lifting right
heel off floor.

Meanwhile, move the
quivering arms forward and
upward with palms facing
forward and fingers pointing
up. Eyes follow arms and
finally gaze up to the front
(Fig. 46).

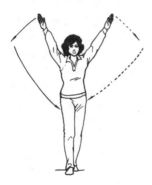

Fig 46

Form 42 Recover Air

With arms still quivering,
bring them down to the sides
while right foot draws up to a
position parallel to and
shoulder-width away from left
foot.

With fingers apart, place
hands over abdomen — left
hand on upper left and right
hand on lower right of navel.
Fingers point in opposite
directions and are a few cm
apart.

Then shake stomach three
times, each time for a few
seconds, with a brief interval in

between. Look straight ahead (Fig. 47).

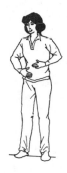

Fig 47

Form 43 Grasp Air

Raise right hand up and out to the front at shoulder level with palm turned down and with thumb and forefinger forming a curve (Fig. 48). Then exert strength to clench fingers into a "hollow fist" leaving a hollow space between fingers and palm.

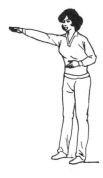

Fig 48

Draw fist back to the front of right part of chest with shoulder relaxed and armpit "empty," and with that part of the fist between thumb and forefinger facing the right *qihu* point. Now you have done your first "grasp air" movement. Look straight ahead.

Raise left hand up and out to the front at shoulder level

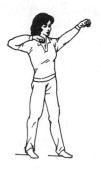

Fig 49

(Fig. 49). Then exert strength to clench fingers into a "hollow fist."

Bend elbow and draw fist back to the front of left part of chest with shoulder relaxed and armpit "empty." That part of the fist between thumb and forefinger faces the left *qihu* point. Look straight ahead.

Alternating the hands, do the "grasp air" movement with feet position unchanged (Fig. 50).

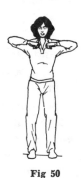

Fig 50

Form 44 Turn Palm and Gather up Air

Rotate right arm outward and reach out hand to the front at shoulder level with palm facing upward. Then exert strength to clench hand into a "hollow fist" and pull fist back to the front of right part of chest with ulnar side facing the right *qihu* point, shoulder relaxed and armpit "empty." Look straight ahead. Now you have "gathered up air" with right hand.

Gather up air with left hand in the same way as described above. Alternating the hands, do the movement five times with feet position unchanged (Fig. 51).

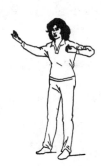

Fig 51

Form 45 Hold Ball

Starting with both hands in front of chest (Fig. 52), raise arms overhead with elbows down, then rotate arms inward and bring them down from both sides in a curve while torso bends forward at about 90 degrees with legs straightened. The *baihui* point at top of head faces downward or forward.

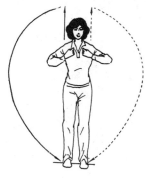

Fig 52

Hang down arms in front of legs with wrists slightly flexed and palms turned up, fingers pointing at each other at about 20 cm apart, as if holding a ball. Look at hands. Feet position unchanged (Fig. 53).

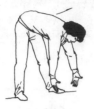

Fig 53

Form 46 Rotate the Ball

Lift up torso slightly and twist to the left while carrying hands to the front left of lower abdomen in a "hold ball" gesture.

Then rotate right arm inward with palm facing down and bring right hand above left hand so that palms face each other at a vertical distance of about 10 cm, still in a "hold ball" gesture. Look at hands.

Imagine yourself rotating the ball with a stroking movement of your arms, wrists and fingers in a clockwise direction (Fig. 54). Coordinate the stroking movement with a rotation of your waist.

Rotate the ball 10 times and stop by the right side of abdomen. Look at hands. Feet position remains unchanged. Knees are slightly bent.

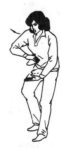

Fig 54

Form 47 Turn Body and Rotate Ball

Rotating both arms simultaneously, bring left hand up and right hand down to turn the ball upside down. Then rotate it with a stroking movement of your arms, wrists and fingers in a counterclockwise direction.

Do the rotating movement eight times while gradually moving the ball to left side of abdomen, turning your waist in coordination (Fig. 55).

Then rotate the ball twice while moving it back to front of abdomen. Meanwhile, turn body back to normal position. Feet position remains unchanged. Look at hands.

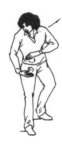

Fig 55

Form 48 Hold Air

Lift up torso and raise arms. Then rotate arms inward and bring hands down to both sides in a curve with legs straightened, torso bending forward with *baihui* point facing forward or downward.

Arms hang down in front of legs with wrists flexed and palms facing upward, fingers separated, thumb and forefinger forming a curve. Fingertips of both hands point at each other, about 30 cm apart, as if holding a bulky weight.

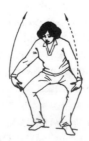

Fig 56

Then bend knees slightly and exert strength to lift the "weight" up to front of chest, arms rotating inward and palms turned inward, while body straightens up. Look ahead to the front. Feet position remains unchanged (Fig. 56).

Form 49 Pass Through Air

With hands still holding the air, raise them up to forehead with palms facing inward, arms rounded, fingers of both hands pointing at each other, about 10 cm apart. Then slowly lower hands down past chest to lower abdomen, where they stay for a few seconds before separating and hanging by the sides. Look straight ahead. Feet position remains unchanged (Fig. 57).

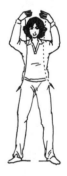

Fig 57

Form 50 Raise Arms

Raise arms out to the front with wrists relaxed and palms facing downward. Then bend elbows and lower them slowly, hands held relaxedly above shoulder level, wrists flexed, elbow tips slightly more than shoulder-width apart. Look straight ahead (Fig. 58).

While sinking elbows, raise hands up again and quickly push palms forward with wrists flexed back, thumbs and forefingers of both hands facing each other, about 10 cm apart.

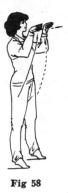

Fig 58

Fingers of both hands point obliquely upward, palms facing forward at forehead level. Look at hands. Feet position remains unchanged (Fig. 59).

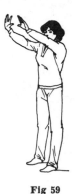

Fig 59

Form 51 Drop Wings

Flex wrists forward in palmar direction and form fingers into claws pointing downward. Look straight ahead. Feet position remains unchanged (Fig. 60).

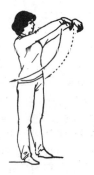

Fig 60

Form 52 Flap Wings to The Back

Bring arms down past hips to the back with elbows bent and forearms lifted up so that the *hegu* point on each hand is pressed against the *shenyu* point. Palms are up, fingers point backward. Look straight ahead. Feet position remains unchanged (Fig. 61).

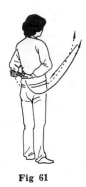

Fig 61

Form 53 Fly Up to One Side

Bring hands down past hips and forward to shoulder level with palms facing downward and fingers pointing forward, elbows slightly bent. Look straight ahead.

Fly up to the left:

Bend right knee and shift weight onto right foot while left foot moves a step forward with knee slightly bent and external side of ball of foot on floor. Meanwhile, press right hand downward and hold it at about 10 cm in front of lower abdomen, with palm facing inward. Four fingers are naturally straight and point to the left, forefinger forming a curve with thumb.

In coordination with movement of right hand, raise left arm to upper left with elbow slightly bent until left

hand comes above head level, palm facing downward and obliquely inward, wrist relaxed, five fingers hanging down naturally, torso twisting slightly to the left. Look at left palm (Fig. 62).

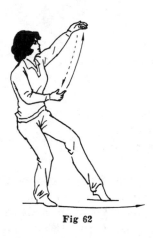

Fig 62

Fly up to the right:

Same as above except that "right" and "left" are reversed (Fig. 63). Do the "flying" movement seven times in the following order: left, right, left, right, left, right, left.

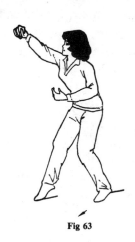

Fig 63

Form 54 Turn Body

After flying up to the left, bring left arm down and right arm up so that both arms extend out to the front, while legs are straightened and body

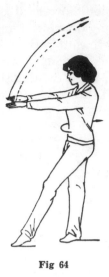

Fig 64

turns back to normal position (Fig. 64).

Then, using both heels as pivot, turn about 180 degrees to the right while arms start to quiver. Look straight ahead.

Form 55 Fly Up to the Sky

While turning body, raise the shaking arms slowly overhead with palms facing forward and fingers pointing up. Now right foot is in front with heel lifted off floor, and weight rests on left foot. Look straight ahead (Fig. 65).

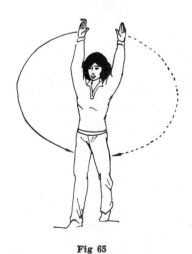

Fig 65

Then lower the quivering arms down to the sides in a curve as shown in Fig. 65.

Form 56 Skim over Water

Left style:

Shift weight onto right foot while left foot moves a step forward with left knee slightly bent and ball of foot on floor.

Meanwhile, bring quivering arms forward and upward to shoulder level. Then, bending right knee sharply, lean torso forward and twist it about 45 degrees to the left while the quivering arms move in a curve to the left.

Left arm goes to upper left until left hand comes above head level with palm facing leftward and thumb pointing obliquely downward, right hand reaching out to front left at chest level with palm turned down. Both arms are naturally bent. Look at left hand (Fig. 66).

Then lift up torso and do "skimming" movement in the right style, which is the same as that of the left style except that "right" and "left" are reversed (Fig. 67).

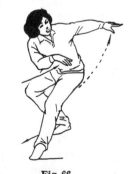

Fig 66

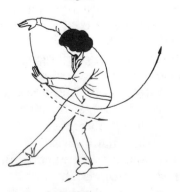

Fig 67

Alternate the two styles in the following order: left, right, left, right, left, right, left.

Form 57 Turn Body

Same as Form 54 (Fig. 64).

Form 58 Fly Upward

Same as Form 55 (Fig. 65).

Form 59 Look for Food

Left style:

Shift weight onto right foot and move left foot a step forward with ball of foot on floor, left leg naturally straightened and right knee deeply bent, torso bending forward.

Move arms from the sides to the front so that they cross in front of left knee. The left arm is on top, left hand points to the right and right hand points to the left. Look down to the front (Fig. 68).

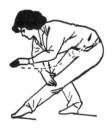

Fig 68

Right style:

Lift up torso a bit and swing arms back to the sides. Shift weight onto left foot and move right foot a step forward (Fig. 69) before proceeding to the right style, which is the same as the left style except that "right" and "left" are reversed.

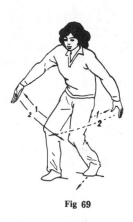

Fig 69

Alternate the two styles in the following order: left, right, left, right, left, right, left.

Form 60 Turn Body

After crossing arms in front of left knee, straighten up torso and stretch right leg while spreading arms and bending elbows so as to lift up forearms with wrists hanging relaxedly in front of abdomen. Palms face downward. Elbows are more than shoulder-width apart. Look straight ahead.

Then, using both heels as pivot, turn around 180 degrees to the right without moving hands. Weight rests on left foot (Fig. 70).

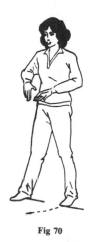

Fig 70

Form 61 Look for the Nest

1. Left style:

Shift weight onto right foot and move left foot a step forward with ball of foot on floor. The torso twists slightly to the left while arms move to left waist side with fingers apart.

The forefinger forms a curve with thumb, fingertips of both hands pointing at each other, a few centimeters apart, palms facing downward.

Then exert strength consciously to flex wrists in a backward direction and press palm down to the side of left hip. Right leg is slightly bent. Look at hands (Fig. 71).

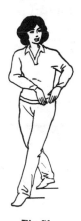

Fig 71

2. Middle style:

Straighten right leg and lift heel off floor while shifting weight onto left foot. Relax wrists and bend elbows. Raise hands up to abdomen while turning torso back to normal position.

Then move right foot a step forward with ball of foot on floor while hands press down to lower abdomen. Left leg is slightly bent. Look at hands.

3. Right style:

Straighten left leg and lift heel off floor while shifting weight onto right foot. Relax wrists and bend elbows while raising hands up to right waist side and twisting torso slightly to the right.

Then move left foot a step forward with ball of foot on floor. Right foot is slightly bent. Exert strength consciously to press hands down to the side of right hip. Look at hands (Fig. 72).

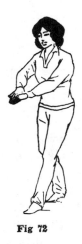

Fig 72

4. Right style:

Shift weight onto left foot and move right foot a step forward. Hands keep pressing down to the side of right hip.

5. Middle style:

Shift weight onto right foot and move left foot a step forward while turning torso back to normal position and pressing hands down to lower abdomen.

6. Left style:

Shift weight onto left foot and move right foot a step forward while pressing hands down to the side of left hip.

7. Middle style:

Shift weight onto right foot and move left foot a step

forward while pressing hands down to lower abdomen (Fig. 73).

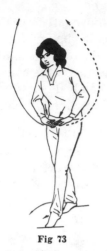

Fig 73

Form 62 Turn Body And Swim

Using left heel as pivot, turn 90 degrees to the left. You are now facing the same direction as you did in Form 1.

While right foot turns in the same direction and moves up half a step to take a parallel stance with left foot, both heels lift slightly off the floor and are about shoulder-width apart.

Meanwhile, quiver arms and move them apart before carrying them upward to a level above forehead. Elbows turn outward, palms face downward and slightly inward. Look straight ahead (Fig. 74).

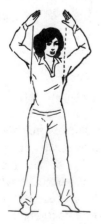

Fig 74

Form 63 Sleep Peacefully and Recover Air

Bring the shaking hands down past face and chest to the front of abdomen. Meanwhile, squat down on both legs with buttocks tucked in and heels lifted off floor. Fingers are separated, forefinger forming a curve with thumb, hands on either side of navel, fingertips pointing toward each other, about 7 cm apart.

Then bend torso slightly forward and lower head with eyes closed (or slightly opened) in meditation for about half a minute, thoughts concentrated on *dantian* point (Fig. 75).

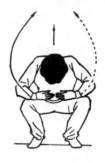

Fig 75

Form 64 Closing Position

Open eyes and rise up slowly with legs straightened and heels on floor, hands slowly raised to

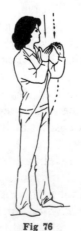

Fig 76

the front of forehead, palms facing inward.

Then slowly bring hands down past chest and abdomen and to the sides (Fig. 76), with internal air sinking down to *dantian*.

Bring right foot to the side of left foot to stand at attention. Look straight ahead (Fig. 77).

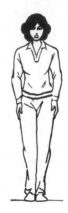

Fig 77

EXERCISES IN 20 FORMS
FOR HEALTH AND LONGEVITY

By WU MINGSHI

Disciple of the late wushu master Wang Ziping

The following set of exercises was compiled by Wang Ziping (1880-1973) in the 1950s. Based on the centuries-old therapeutic exercises of daoyin, wuqinxi, yijinjing, and baduanjin, it involves both qigong (breathing exercises) and movements of the body. Regular practice of this set of exercises has proved effective in curing many chronic ailments, including pains in the neck, shoulders, waist and legs, as well as cardiovascular diseases.

During the past two decades and more, it has been practiced by thousands upon thousands of people, especially by elderly and middle-aged people. Wang Ziping himself also exercised it regularly in his old age. The fact that he lived to 93 shows that this set of exercises is well worth the name of "longevity."

Here are some points for attention:

1. Persist in doing the exercises if you want to benefit from them. As a Chinese proverb says, "Small gains in 100 days and big gains in 1,000 days."

2. Repeat each form 6-36 times. Practice twice a day, morning and evening, 30-60 minutes each time. Increase the amount of exercise gradually, in keeping with your health condition and as long as you don't feel uncomfortable or overtired.

3. Concentrate your mind on the movements. Breathe evenly and use abdominal respiration as time goes by.

4. Exercise in a place where the air is fresh, but not in a strong draft.

5. Do some cooling-down exercises at the end of each session. These include wrist-rotation, arm swings, pats on arms, chest, buttocks and thighs, and massage on cheeks and from temples up to the top of head and down to the nape. Or just take a walk.

**Form 1   Get out the Stale and
            Take in the Fresh**

A. Stand upright with feet shoulder-width apart, right palm on abdomen and left palm on the back of right hand (Fig. 1).

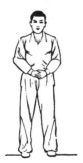

Fig 1

B. Breathe deeply and slowly, with tip of tongue touching palate. Keep body relaxed, head erect and eyes naturally closed.

**Form 2   Nestlings Receive
            Food**

A. Stand upright with feet shoulder-width apart, arms hanging at sides.

B. Raise both hands to the front of chest, palms facing down and fingers of one hand pointing at those of the other (Fig. 2).

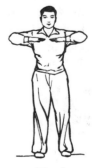

Fig 2

C. Press palms slowly downward until arms are almost straight (Fig. 3). Inhale and apply force to shoulders when raising hands. Exhale and relax shoulders when pressing palms down.

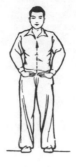

Fig 3

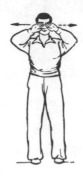

Fig 5

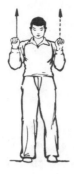

Fig 7

Form 3　The Roc Presses Its Crop

A. Stand upright with feet shoulder-width apart, right palm on chest and left palm on the back of right hand.

B. Move palms in circles — first clockwise and then counter-clockwise — to massage chest, the upper part of abdomen and the area around navel lightly. Breathe once with every circling movement. Eyes look up (Fig. 4). Keep head slightly raised and torso erect.

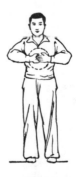

Fig 4

Form 4　Draw the Bow on Both Sides

A. Stand upright with feet shoulder-width apart. Raise hands to eye level, palms facing outward, fingers slightly bent and elbows pointing obliquely forward (Fig. 5).

B. Separate hands horizontally until forearms are vertical, palms loosely clenched. chest is thrown out as far as possible (Fig. 6).

C. Return hands to original position with chest drawn in. Inhale when separating hands and exhale when drawing them back.

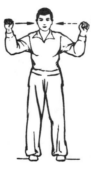

Fig 6

Form 5　The King Lifts A Tripod

A. Stand upright with feet shoulder-width apart. Clench both hands loosely as you raise them slowly to the front of shoulders (Fig. 7).

B. Open both hands as you raise them slowly overhead, palms up. Eyes follow hands (Fig. 8).

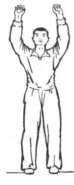

Fig 8

C. Clench both hands loosely as you lower them to the front of the shoulders, applying a little force to fingers. Inhale when raising hands and exhale when lowering them.

Form 6　Raise Arms to Pluck Fruit

A. Stand upright with feet shoulder-width apart, arms hanging at sides.

B. Raise left hand along body, palm facing inward, and rotate it forward and up when it is overhead, arm fully stretched. Heels are slightly raised and eyes follow hand. At the same time, raise right hand along lower back, palm facing outward (Figs. 9-10).

C. Place left hand behind back and right hand beside right waist. Repeat the movements in B, reversing right

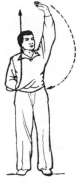

Fig 9

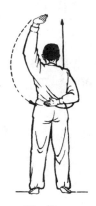

Fig 10

and left. Inhale when raising hands and exhale when lowering them.

Form 7 Search the Sea Bottom

A. Stand upright with feet shoulder-width apart, arms akimbo.

B. Crane neck and look down about two meters away, first to the right and then to the left, breathing once with every body turn (Figs. 11a-b).

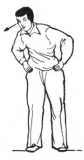

Fig 11a

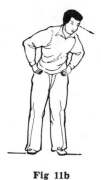

Fig 11b

Form 8 The Rhino Looks At the Moon

A. Stand upright with feet shoulder-width apart, arms akimbo.

B. Turn head to right and left as backward as possible and look up, breathing once with every turn (Figs. 12a-b).

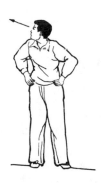

Fig 12a

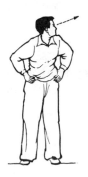

Fig 12b

Do not turn torso. Keep chin slightly drawn in.

Form 9 Lotus Leaves Sway In the Wind

A. Stand upright with feet a bit wider apart than shoulders. Rub palm on the other hand's back before placing them on hips, thumbs pointing forward.

B. Massage back forcibly with both hands down to buttocks (Fig. 13).

C. Circle hips clockwise and counter-clockwise, enlarging the circles gradually and keeping torso erect (Fig. 14).

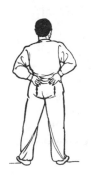

Fig 13

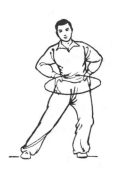

Fig 14

Form 10 Push a Stone Tablet

A. Stand upright with feet a bit wider apart than shoulders. Arms hang at sides.

B. Clench left hand as you place it on left hip. Turn torso to the left and push right hand forward at shoulder level, with palm facing forward, head

turned to look backward
(Fig. 15a).

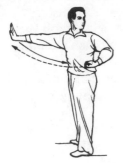

Fig 15a

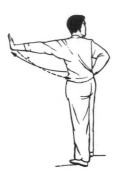

Fig 15b

C. Repeat the movements in B, reversing right and left (Fig. 15b).

Inhale when pushing hand forward and exhale when drawing it back. Apply a little force to wrist. Do not move feet or stiffen arms. Increase the degrees of body turn as time goes on.

Form 11 Insert Palm into Mt. Huashan

A. Stand upright with feet a bit wider apart than shoulders, arms hanging at sides.

B. Turn body to the left and take a left bow stance — with left leg bent at knee and right leg straightened, heel on floor. At the same time, move left hand forward and, with palm turned down, withdraw it in a circular movement to waist side. The right hand thrusts forward, palm facing leftward as if you were stabbing with a

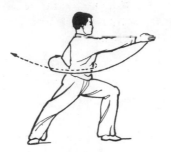

Fig 16a

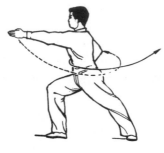

Fig 16b

knife. Eyes follow right hand (Fig. 16a).

C. Repeat the movements in B, reversing right and left (Fig. 16b).

Form 12 Part the Mane on A White Horse

A. Stand upright with feet shoulder-width apart, hands crossed in front of abdomen.

B. Bend forward, eyes looking at hands (Fig. 17).

C. Straighten up and raise crossed hands overhead, with

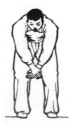

Fig 17

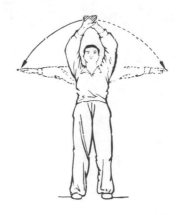

Fig 18

torso fully stretched. Extend arms sideways, looking first at left hand and then at right hand (Fig. 18).

D. Return to starting position. Inhale when raising hands and exhale when lowering them.

Form 13 The Phoenix Spreads Its Wings

A. Stand upright with feet a bit wider apart than shoulders, arms hanging at sides.

B. Bend forward with knees slightly flexed as you raise left hand slowly in a sideward curve, while right palm presses left knee lightly, head turned up to look at left hand (Fig. 19a).

C. Raise right hand slowly, while left palm presses right

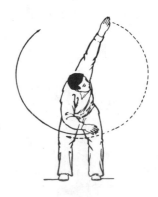

Fig 19a

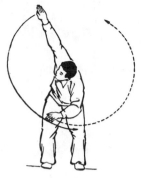

Fig 19b

knee lightly, head turned up to look at right hand (Fig. 19b). Inhale when turning up head and exhale when turning it to the front.

Form 14 The Carpenter Handles a Drill

A. Stand upright with feet shoulder-width apart, hands clenched into fists at waist sides.

B. Turn body to the right and drop into a semi-squat, left knee pressed against right calf. At the same time, thrust left fist forward at shoulder level (Fig. 20a).

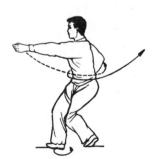

Fig 20a

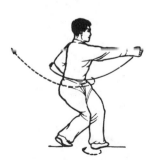

Fig 20b

C. Repeat the movements in B, reversing right and left (Fig. 20b).

This exercise may be difficult to elderly people. They can skip it at the initial stage.

Form 15 The Black Dragon Turns Around

A. Stand upright with feet a bit wider apart than shoulders, arms hanging at sides.

B. Turn body to the left for a left bow stance as you clench left hand into fist at waist and push right palm forward (Fig. 21).

C. Open left hand and move it sideways as you turn right hand downward. Move both palms clockwise in two circles, eyes following hands (Figs. 22a-d).

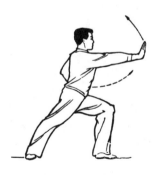

Fig 21

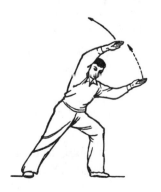

Fig 22a (side view)

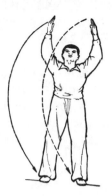

Fig 22b (side view)

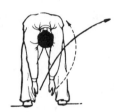

Fig 22c (side view)

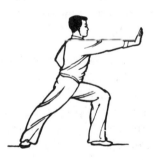

Fig 22d

D. Repeat the movements in B, reversing right and left and moving both hands counter-clockwise.

Breathe once with every circling movement. Keep both legs straight when circling hands.

Form 16 The Arhat Subdues A Tiger

A. Stand upright with feet a bit wider apart than shoulders, arms akimbo.

B. Bend left and right knees alternately, eyes looking straight ahead (Figs. 23a-b).

Inhale when bending knee and exhale when straightening it. Keep torso erect. Bend knee slightly at the initial stage.

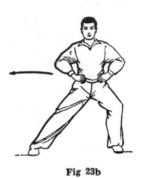

Fig 23a

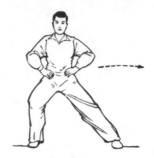

Fig 23b

Form 17 The White Crane Circles Its Knees

A. Stand upright with feet together and knees slightly bent. Massage knees gently with palms separately, eyes looking down ahead (Fig. 24).

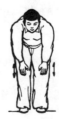

Fig 24

B. Circle knees several times, first clockwise and then counter-clockwise, enlarging the circles gradually and breathing

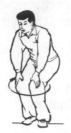

Fig 25

once with every circling movement (Fig. 25).

Form 18 The Friar Sits on His Haunches

A. Stand upright with feet shoulder-width apart, hands clenched at waist.

B. Squat down with both arms extended forward (Fig. 26).

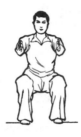

Fig 26

C. Return to starting position.

Inhale when bending knees and exhale when standing up. Keep torso erect. The depth of squats is to be determined by yourself.

Form 19 Kick Lower Legs in Four Directions

A. Stand upright with feet together and arms akimbo.

B. Raise left knee and kick lower leg forward, toes pointed (Fig. 27 — side view). Set foot down. Repeat seven times.

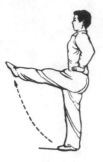

Fig 27

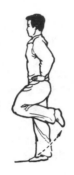

Fig 28

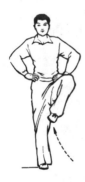

Fig 29

C. Kick left lower leg backward, so that heel touches right buttock, if possible (Fig. 28 — side view). Set foot down. Repeat seven times.

D. Repeat the movements in B and C with right leg.

E. Raise left knee and kick lower leg inward (Fig. 29). Set foot down. Repeat seven times.

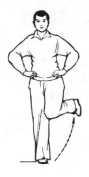

Fig 30

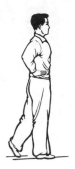

Fig 32

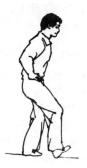

Fig 35

F. Raise left knee and kick lower leg outward (Fig. 30). Set foot down. Repeat seven times.

G. Repeat the movements in E and F with right leg.

Inhale when kicking lower leg and exhale when setting foot down. Kicks should not be too forceful. Keep torso and head erect, eyes looking forward.

Form 20   The Fairy Steps Back and Forth

A. Stand upright with heels together and arms akimbo.

B. Take a step forward with left foot in heel-to-toe motion (Fig. 31).

D. Take a step backward with right foot in a toe-to-heel motion. Shift weight onto right leg and raise toes of left foot as much as possible (Fig. 33).

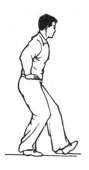

Fig 33

E. Place left sole flat on floor. Take a step forward with right foot and another with left foot in toe-to-heel motion (Fig. 34).

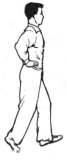

Fig 31

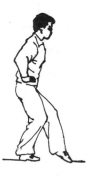

Fig 34

C. Take a step forward with right foot, shifting weight onto right leg and raising left heel as much as possible (Fig. 32).

F. Take a step backward with left foot in toe-to-heel motion, shifting weight onto left leg and raising toes of

right foot as much as possible (Fig. 35).

Breathe once with every step taken, eyes looking ahead.

69

SEVEN-STAR BOXING OF HU MEICHENG

Hu Meiching, 75, is an adviser to the National Qigong Research Society. He started learning Chinese martial arts at the age of 17, taking six masters as his teachers as he pursued his studies over the years.

On the basis of several ancient forms of fitness and breathing exercises, including taijiquan, baduanjin, and the five-animal play, he has worked out a set of exercises called "Seven-Star Boxing," which has been adopted by qigong training classes with satisfactory results. The seven forms are composed of graceful, well-balanced movements done in a continuous flow and involve every movable joint of the body.

Proceeding from the principle of combining meditation (internal work) with action (external work), the exercises are aimed at promoting circulation and improving the network of channels in the human body through which vital energy circulates and along which the acupuncture points are distributed.

Seven-Star Boxing has proved effective in varying degrees in curing such chronic ailments as strains in the limbs, rheumarthritis, heart diseases, hypertension, tuberculosis, tracheitis, pulmonary emphysema, hepatitis, gastric diseases, and neurasthenia.

Exercisers should bear the following points in mind:

1. Movements should be continuous. Coordinate the movements of the body and the limbs. Breathe evenly.

2. Concentrate your mind on the dantian, an acupuncture point about 5 cm below the navel.

3. Relax yourself.

4. Sufferers from the aforementioned ailments should refrain from intense exercise at the beginning. Those with hypertension and heart diseases should not bend the trunk too low. Stop the exercise if it makes you feel unwell.

Commencing Form

Stand upright and move left foot sideways so that your feet are a bit more than shoulder-width apart, toes pointing slightly inward. Arms hang naturally on both sides and eyes look down ahead. Rid your mind of all stray thoughts (Figs. 1-2).

Relax yourself — first loosen up the acupuncture point of *yintang* between the eyebrows, then the point of *renzhong* in the middle of the philtrum, with corners of mouth raised a bit as if you were wearing a smile. Then loosen your shoulders and whole body.

Words of command:
Attention — Side step — Relax.

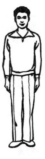

Fig 1

Fig 2

Form 1   Draw the Bow on Both Sides

This is an exercise for bending and stretching the arms.

1. Turn body to left on both heels, with left leg stretched and right leg flexed and buttocks lowered. As you turn body, bend arms slightly, clench hands into fists and bring them together back to back (Fig. 3).

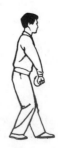

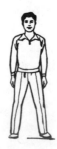

Fig 3

Words of command: Turn to left — Clench fists.

2. Raise fists to the front of chest and move left foot a little backward, toes on floor, for an empty stance, most of weight on right foot (Fig. 4).

Words of command: Raise Fists — Empty stance.

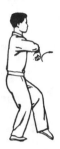

Fig 4

3. Open fists and turn palms up (Fig. 5). Draw hands to the back and lift left foot as you take in a deep breath (Fig. 6). Raise hands overhead from behind the back, turning palms forward as you slowly breathe out.

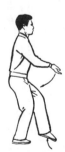

Fig 5

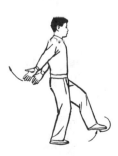

Fig 6

At the same time, circle left sole clockwise with ankle joint as the hinge before taking a step forward. Heel lands first to form a left bow stance, with rear leg stretched and front leg flexed at knee (Fig. 7). Bend trunk forward (Fig. 8).

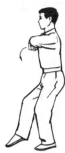

Fig 7

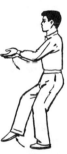

Fig 8

4. Straighten up trunk and withdraw left foot a bit while pulling hands back. At the same time turn about to the right 180 degrees on both heels (Figs. 9-10).

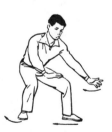

Fig 9

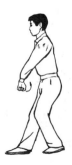

Fig 10

Repeat movements in 1, 2, 3, reversing right and left (Figs. 11-15). Then straighten up trunk and withdraw left foot a bit while pulling hands back (Fig. 16).

Words of command: Withdraw foot — Turn About — Then repeat the actions in 1, 2, 3.

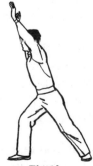

Fig 11

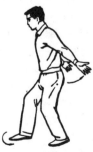

Fig 12

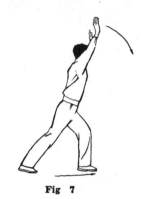

Fig 13

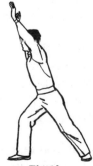

Fig 14

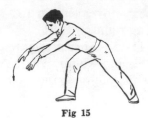

Fig 15

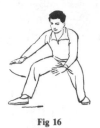

Fig 16

Form 2   Stand Firm and Support Sky

This is an exercise involving the exertion of strength by the extremities in an upward or downward direction.

1. Turn toes of right foot inward and move it a bit towards left foot, turning body to the left and drawing both hands to the front, palms up (Fig. 17). Turn over palms and clench them into fists (Fig. 18).

Words of command: Turn left — Turn over palms — Clench fists.

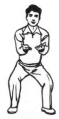

Fig 17

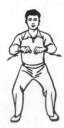

Fig 18

2. Open fists and place hands besides ribs, fingers pointing down (Fig. 19). Drop hands on both sides as you squat down slowly until thighs are parallel with ground (Figs. 20a-b).

Words of command: Hands down — Squat.

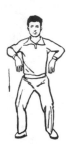

Fig 19

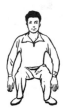

Fig 20a

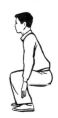

Fig 20b

3. Point fingers forward (Figs. 21a-b).

Words of command: Palms down.

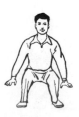

Fig 21a

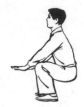

Fig 21b

4. Lift hands up to shoulder level with palms facing forward (Fig. 22). Stretch arms overhead with palms up as you rise to full stature on toes, taking a deep breath at the same time (Fig. 23).

Words of Command: Rise — Stretch arms — Stand on toes — Inhale — Exhale.

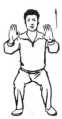

Fig 22

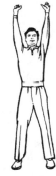

Fig 23

Form 3   Move Heaven and Earth

This is a turning exercise around the longitudinal axis of the body, with a maximum twist of the head, neck, waist, and legs.

1. Set heels on ground and move hands down to left side as

if you were holding a ball (henceforth referred to as hold-ball gesture), right hand on top (Fig. 24).

At the same time, turn torso and knees to the left with left knee slightly flexed. Then turn to the right with right knee slightly flexed and take a hold-ball gesture on right side, left hand on top (Fig. 25).

Words of command: Heels down — Hold ball.

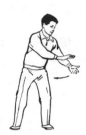

Fig 24

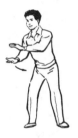

Fig 25

2. Shift weight onto left leg as you turn torso to the left on heels, hands still in hold-ball gesture (Fig. 26). Move right hand under left elbow as if you were rolling the ball with your palms.

Meanwhile, turn about to the left 180 degrees with legs crossed and toes of both feet turned toward each other to form a triangle (Figs. 27a-b). Move left hand downward and backward and right hand upward and forward, with arms curved and spread (Fig. 28).

"Flash" right palm by moving right hand past forehead to overhead position, palm facing forward, while left

hand moves to the back, palm facing backward (Figs. 29a-b).

Words of command: Turn left — Roll ball — Flash palm.

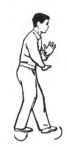

Fig 26

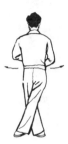

Fig 27a

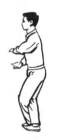

Fig 27b

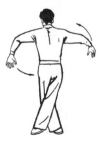

Fig 28

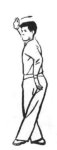

Fig 29a

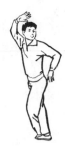

Fig 29b

3. Turn about to the right 180 degrees on heels. Bend trunk to right side as far as possible as you lower right hand from the back of head and reach down towards the ground, while left hand is raised overhead. Both palms face forward. Right leg slightly flexed at knee and left leg fully stretched (Figs. 30-31).

Words of command: Turn about — Bend to the right.

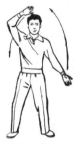

Fig 30

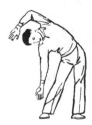

Fig 31

4. Form a hold-ball gesture on right side with left hand on top (Fig. 32). Turn to the left and form a hold-ball gesture with right hand on top while shifting weight onto left leg

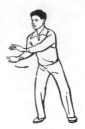

Fig 32

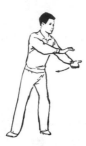

Fig 33

(Fig. 33). Repeat movements in 2 and 3, reversing right and left (Figs. 34-39).

Words of command: Hold ball — Turn right — Then repeat as in 2 and 3, reversing left and right.

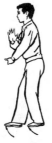

Fig 34

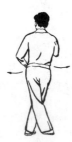

Fig 35a

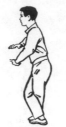

Fig 35b

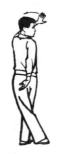

Fig 36

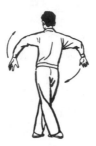

Fig 37a

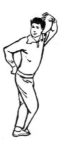

Fig 37b

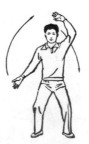

Fig 38

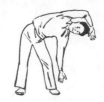

Fig 39

Form 4 Bend Forward and Backward

This is a bending exercise, with the body leaning forward as much as possible.

1. Straighten up and spread arms with elbows a little bent, palms down (Fig. 40).

Words of commands: Straighten up — Spread arms.

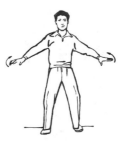

Fig 40

2. Move both hands in a horizontal circle that goes backward and outward and then forward and inward under armpits until they come out to the front of abdomen, palms up, and then cross them in front of chest, palms turned inward, right palm on the back of left palm (Figs. 41-42).

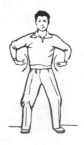

Fig 41

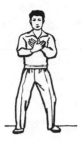

Fig 42

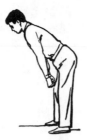

Fig 44c

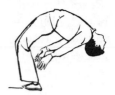

Fig 46b

Words of command: Circle hands — Cross palms.

3. Rotate forearms internally and clench hands into fists before separating them, arms rounded (Fig. 43). Bend trunk forward as much as possible so as to bring backs of fists in touch with heels. Look backward through legs (Figs. 44a-b).

Beginners, aged people, and those of weak constitution may just bend slightly forward with hands reaching knees (Fig. 44c).

Words of command: Rotate arms — Clench fists — Bend forward.

4. Straighten up and open arms at a level slightly lower than shoulders while opening fists and turning palms downward (Fig. 45). Bend backward as much as possible, with hands hanging on both sides (Figs. 46a-b).

Words of command: Straighten up — Open arms — Bend backward.

Form 5 The Roc Spreads Its Wings

This is a stretching exercise with arms and legs fully extended at an angle of 45 degrees with ground.

1. Straighten up and form a hold-ball gesture with right hand on top (Fig. 47).

Words of command: Straighten up — Hold ball.

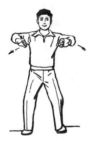

Fig 43

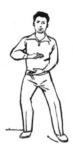

Fig 47

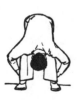

Fig 44a

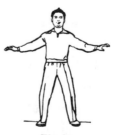

Fig 45

2. Shift weight onto right leg while lifting left foot and rotating its sole clockwise around the ankle joint (Fig. 48).

Words of command: Lift foot — Rotate sole.

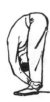

Fig 44b

Fig 46a

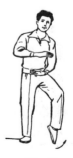

Fig 48

3. Form "sword-fingers" with both hands by bending the ring and little fingers, extending the middle and index fingers and pressing thumb on ring finger.

Raise left hand and lower right hand so that the arms form a straight line slanting at an angle of 45 degrees with ground.

Reach out with the "sword-fingers" to the fullest extent. Left palm faces backward and right palm faces forward.

At the same time, stretch left leg and draw it across right leg from behind, placing the little and fourth toes on ground.

Keep trunk erect and left leg parallel to right arm. Look first at left hand and then at right hand (Fig. 49).

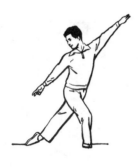

Fig 49

Words of command: Stretch leg — Spread wings.

4. Move left foot back to left side of right foot and form a hold-ball gesture with left hand on top (Fig. 50). Repeat

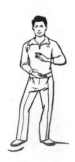

Fig 50

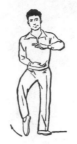

Fig 51

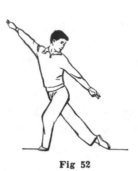

Fig 52

movements in 2 and 3, reversing right and left (Figs. 51-52).

Words of command: Recover foot — Hold ball — Then repeat as in 2 and 3.

Form 6   Scale

This is a balancing exercise, with trunk, hands and one leg forming a horizontal line.

1. Place hands in front of ribs with palms up and recover right foot to the normal stance (Fig. 53).

Words of command: Recover foot.

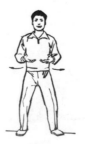

Fig 53

2. Move left foot a step backward and shift weight onto left leg, which is bent at knee, while keeping right leg straight.

At the same time straighten arms by lowering forearms down and out to the sides with palms facing forward (Figs. 54a-b).

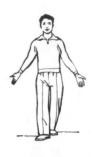

Fig 54a

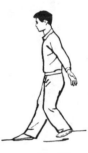

Fig 54b

Words of command: Step back — Bend leg — Straighten arms.

3. Shift weight onto right leg. Bend right leg and straighten left leg while spreading arms (Fig. 55).

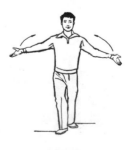

Fig 55

4. Bring lower part of left leg up to the back of thigh with ankle plantar-flexed. Form sword-fingers with both hands and bring them up to the side of ears (Fig. 56).

Words of command: Fold leg — Bend arms — Point ears (with sword-fingers).

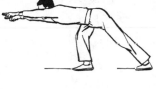

Fig 57c

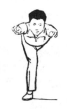

Fig 59b

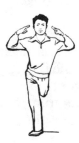

Fig 56

Beginners, aged people, and those with weak constitution may keep rear foot on ground (Fig. 57c) before trying to raise leg progressively to the horizontal level.

Words of command: Extend arms — Stretch leg.

6. Pull hands back to the front of chest with palms down and set left foot down beside right foot (Fig. 58). Repeat movements in 2-5, reversing right and left (Figs. 59a-62b).

Words of command: Withdraw hand — Recover foot — Repeat as in 2-5.

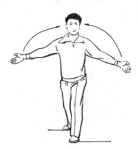

Fig 60

5. Bend trunk forward, stretching left leg backward and extending both arms forward so that they form a horizontal line. Concentrate your mind on fingertips and toes. Raise head and look ahead (Figs. 57a-b).

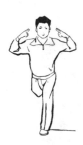

Fig 61

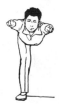

Fig 57a

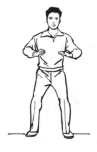

Fig 58

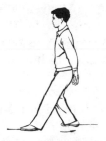

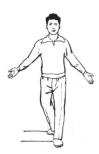

Fig 62a

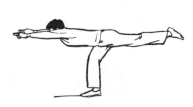

Fig 57b

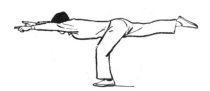

Fig 59a

Fig 62b

Form 7   The Heaven Revolves

In this exercise you turn your trunk and arms in big circles.

1. Set right foot down beside left foot to form a horse-ride stance as you pull your hands back to the front of chest with palms down (Fig. 63).

Words of command: Recover foot — Withdraw hands.

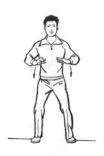

Fig 63

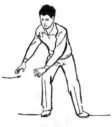

Fig 64

2. Bend forward and move hands down to right side (Fig. 64). Forming "sword-fingers" with both hands, swing your arms and trunk leftward, backward, rightward and forward in a big circle (Figs. 65-71).

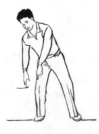

Fig 65

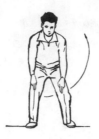

Fig 66

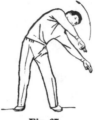

Fig 67

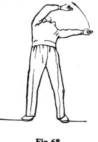

Fig 68

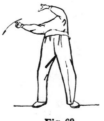

Fig 69

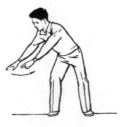

Fig 70

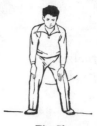

Fig 71

Words of command: Bend trunk — Sword-fingers — Circle.

3. Move sword-fingered hands to left side. Open them and form sword-fingers again before circling trunk and arms in the other direction (Figs. 72-78).

Words of command: Open hands — Sword-fingers — Circle.

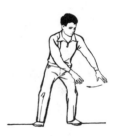

Fig 72

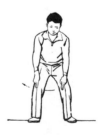

Fig 73

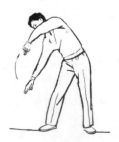

Fig 74

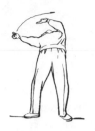

Fig 75

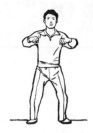

Fig 79

Closing Form

Open fists and lower them to waist side (Fig. 80). At the same time, straighten trunk and legs slowly to return to the commencing position (Fig. 81).

Words of command: Open fists — Arms down — Straighten legs — Recover.

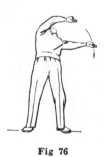

Fig 76

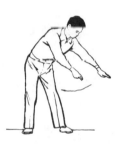

Fig 77

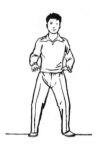

Fig 80

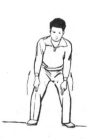

Fig 78

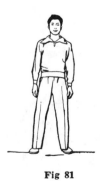

Fig 81

4. Straighten up. Clench hands into fists and raise them to the front of chest (Fig. 79).

Words of command: Straighten up — Raise fists.

TEN-MINUTE QIGONG EXERCISE

By ZHUAN ZAI

Researcher, Beijing Qigong Society

In this bustling world of ours, many people feel the need for fitness training, but are often hard pressed for time. Here is a simple qigong exercise which may answer their needs. It just takes 10 minutes or so to go through the whole course, and it can be done anywhere and at any time you want.

At first you will need a quiet place where you can concentrate on the exercise, but once you get used to it you can practice in a noisy environment without being distracted.

The exercise is done in the following way:

1. Posture

You may adopt any of three body positions — standing, sitting, or lying. Choose the one that makes you feel most comfortable and relaxed so that you can concentrate on your exercise.

A. Standing position. Stand with feet shoulder-width apart, knees slightly flexed and turned inward as if gripping a basketball. Adjust the intensity of exercise by altering the degree of knee flexion.

Bend arms and raise hands in front of chest, with palms facing each other and fingers slightly apart.

Arms should be rounded, shoulders lowered and elbows down — just as if you were ready to catch a basketball tossed to you.

B. Sitting position. You may sit with your torso erect or in an inclined position, and with your hands and knees held in the same way as in the standing posture. Adjust the intensity of exercise by altering the position of your arms.

The farther you hold your arms out to the front, the greater the intensity of exercise. If you find holding the arms out too tiring, you may draw your upper arms to a vertical position and hold the forearms level in front of you.

C. Lying position. Doing the exercise in this position before going to sleep is most effective in curing insomnia. Hold up your arms with palms facing each other and fingers slightly apart. If you are strong enough, you may reach your hands until your arms form an obtuse angle with your body. Hold your hands shoulder-width apart.

Only when you have practiced to the point where subconscious movements are activated by your qi should your arms be spread farther apart, which will make the exercise more strenuous.

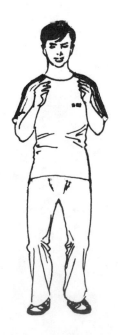

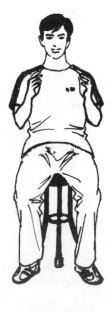

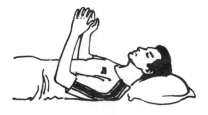

Lying position.

Standing position.

Sitting position.

You are said to open your palms when you draw them away from each other and close them when you bring them closer together. The same is said of the movements of your knees in the sitting posture. The opening and closing movements are graded as large, small, and slight, according to the degree to which the palms or knees are separated or brought towards each other.

When there is no movement of the palms or knees, they are said to be in a static position. The movements of the palms and those of the knees should be done separately or alternately so that you won't have to divide your attention.

2. Mental activity

A. Mental replay: Go over your opening and closing movements in your mind. That is the basic aspect of your mental activity that makes your exercise effective.

B. Visionary resistance: Imagine that between your palms or knees there is a highly resilient balloon or spring or rubber band that offers resistance to your opening and closing movements. Such mental activity calls for a coordination between the sensory and motor nerves and stimulates the flow of qi in your system.

An opening or closing movement may be done over a large range lasting as long as one breath, or over a smaller range that coincides with a heart beat in duration. Start with larger movements and then gradually shorten the range while deepening your concentration until you can feel the slightest movement.

In due course you will enter into a state of complete tranquility. Then you can start thinking of the opening and closing movements while your palms and knees remain in a static condition. At this stage you are physically immobile but mentally active.

During the exercise, you may synchronize your movements with mental activity, so that when you open your palms you imagine that they were being forced to "close" by a magnet or a rubber band, and when you "close" them you get the feeling as if they were being repulsed — or opened — by a magnet or an air mass.

Also, when doing a "large" opening movement, you should imagine yourself doing several closing moves in the process. Likewise, a large closing movement should be punctuated with thoughts about opening movements.

In this way, you will feel halts in your movements and movements in your halts. As you visualize opening or closing movements at the in-

stant of immobility, you will have a growing sensation of the flow of qi in your system, which activates the involuntary movements of your palms. You should start with your palm movements, and only when you regularly experience the sensation of qi should you go on to practice with your knees.

Those who have a headache or feel dizzy should not overstrain themselves with mental effort and their attention should be mainly directed to the performance of the opening and closing movements.

For those suffering from insomnia or gastrointestinal diseases, it is beneficial to do the exercise in the lying position before going to sleep. First do the palm movements in combination with mental activity.

When you feel a strong sensation of qi in you, put down your palms slowly and place them on your lower abdomen. Then concentrate your thoughts on the dantian, the point about 5 cm below the navel.

Qigong exercise involving knee movement will help alleviate or cure palpitation. Persistent practice will help lower blood pressure in those suffering from hypertension.

QIGONG THERAPY: SIMPLE METHODS

By WAI GAO

Editor, China Qigong Journal

1. Deep Breathing Exercise for Health Promotion

Before exercising, sit down quietly for a few minutes and clear your mind of all thoughts. Then close your eyes and relax and mentally direct your attention to dantian, a point about 5 cm below your navel, while using your nose (your mouth is shut) to inhale slowly. Imagine yourself drawing the breath down to dantian and holding it there for half a minute. This may be prolonged progressively for as much as two or three minutes.

Now make an effort to pull your navel as inward as possible for about one minute before allowing it to return to its normal position. Then follows the process of exhalation, which should come naturally and without any conscious effort. This means that you must give no thought to your breathing and must direct all your attention to dantian, imagining yourself looking at and listening to it all this while.

A practice session may last 20 minutes at the outset and be gradually lengthened to a maximum of 60 minutes. Walk around for 50 or 60 steps after each session. At least two sessions are required every day.

The exercise can be done in either sitting or supine position. It must be done daily without interruption to produce the desired effect. By the third month you will start feeling warm and comfortable after doing the exercise. Years of regular practice will keep you fit and help prolong your life.

2. Exercise for Curing Gastroptosis

Lie down on your back with your knees bent at about 115 degrees, both feet lightly propped against the back of the bed, buttocks raised to a height of about 5 cm, arms naturally stretched, palms down, and with a pillow beneath your head (see diagram).

Relax your whole body. Applying abdominal respiration, draw a deep breath slowly and gently while placing your tongue on the hard palate. Then exhale slowly with your tongue detached from the palate. Close your eyes relaxedly and direct your attention to dantian.

The exercise should be done three or four times a day, each time lasting 30 to 60 minutes. Diet yourself properly. Feed on easily digestible food. Have more meals a day and eat sparingly for each meal.

3. Ear Exercise for Curing Chronic Otitis Media

A. Clean your ears with cotton swabs before the exercise.

B. You may either sit or stand when doing the exercise. In any case you must keep calm and relaxed. Put your palms over your ears and rub them in a circular movement for a hundred times. The rubbing should be forceful enough to produce a sensation of heat in your ears. There should be some hollow space between the palm and the earhole lest the pressure of the palm should hurt your ear.

C. With a rubbing motion of the palm, fold the auricle of each ear over the external auditory meatus and keep it there with the part of your palm where it meets with the base of the fingers. Then place the forefinger over the middle finger and snap it down on the mastoidal bone behind the ear. Repeat this for a hundred times.

D. Do the exercise once every morning. Generally it will take effect in a week's time but to consolidate the effect you must go on practicing a long time.

4. Teeth Clenching Exercise

Holding your breath and clenching your teeth while urinating will not only help keep your teeth firm and healthy; it will also help strengthen your kidneys and add to your vital energy.

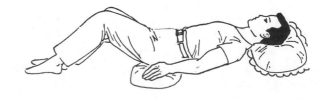

QIGONG CURES SEMINAL EMISSION

By HU BIN

Professor, Beijing College of Traditional Chinese Medicine

There are two kinds of seminal emission, physiological and pathological. Seminal emission once every one or two weeks is quite normal for adolescents and adults. If it occurs several times a week, it should be considered a disease and must be treated in time, and any delay may lead to nervous breakdown, dizziness, tinnitus, poor memory, distraction, inertia, palpitation, shortness of breath or backache.

Seminal emission is mostly caused by neurasthenia, oversleeping, overtiredness, soft bedding, sleeping in prone position or reading of pornography. Athletes should guard against seminal emission before competition because it will affect their performances. Our clinic experience proves qigong to be effective in preventing and curing seminal emission.

The Exercises

Before doing the exercises, relieve yourself in the toilet, loosen your clothes and belt and choose a quiet room with fresh air.

Cushion one end of the bed, making it about three inches higher than the other end. Or just sit on a pillow. A hard board bed is preferable to a spring mattress.

Sit upright at the higher end of the bed, facing the lower end, legs held straight forward with toes pointing upward, palms on knees (Fig. 1). Close fingers and pull fists to your sides, drawing elbows as backward as possible (Fig. 2).

Open both hands with palms facing upward and begin to inhale. Draw in abdomen and raise hands past ears as if lifting a weight until they reach the limit. At the same time, contract rectum and interlace fingers above head, palms up. Look up at the back of hands.

Then start to exhale (Fig. 3). Lower head and lean forward. Meanwhile, stretch out both arms forward and touch toes with fingers (Fig. 4). Then return to the original upright sitting position. Repeat this 10 times to begin with and add two reps every day until the daily quota reaches 70 by the end of the first month. Keep to this figure henceforth.

Exercise twice a day, after getting up and before going to bed. Usually, satisfactory results will be achieved after two months practice. For an athlete a daily quota of 20 reps is sufficient to prevent seminal emission.

Points to Remember

1. While touching toes, both legs must be held straight. This may be a bit difficult for a beginner. But he will be able to do it after more practice.

2. Start to breathe in when hands are opened. Inhalation should be slow and continuous.

3. Contract rectum while raising hands.

4. Breathe out slowly and steadily when bending forward.

5. Sit calmly for 10 minutes after the exercise.

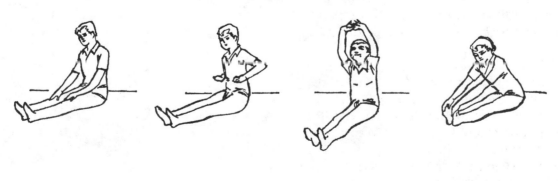

Fig 1   Fig 2   Fig 3   Fig 4

STANDING EXERCISE: A BASIC SKILL

By QIN QINGFENG

Head Coach, Wushu, Beijing University

The "Neijing," a book on internal medicine written more than 2,000 years ago, recommends "stand still and enter meditation" as a means of keeping fit. One of the proverbs in common use today in the wushu community says: "Do the standing exercise before you start the routine proper." Another says, "A performer with a poor standing position is just like a house without pillars."

Every wushu school has its own standing postures which form the basis of all movements.

A standing posture can also be practiced independently as a fitness exercise. Being easy to learn and suitable for people of all ages, this kind of exercise enjoys wide popularity across the country.

Following are eight standing postures commonly practiced today:

1. Ride-horse posture of the Shaolin School (Fig. 1)

Stand firmly with feet parallel to each other and about three times the length of your foot apart. Squat down until thighs are almost horizontal, with toes of both feet turned slightly inward and purchasing the ground. Knees are turned outward and in a vertical line with toes.

Body weight is equally distributed on legs. Hold arms round in front at shoulder level, palms facing down. Middle fingers point at each other and all fingers slightly spread out. Look at the space between middle fingers with half-closed eyes.

2. On Guard posture of the Shaolin School (Fig. 2)

Take a left empty stance with left foot in front, toes turned about 15 degrees inward. Trunk is turned slightly to the left, with 70 percent of the body weight on right foot, which is about 60 cm from and parallel to left foot, all toes press on ground.

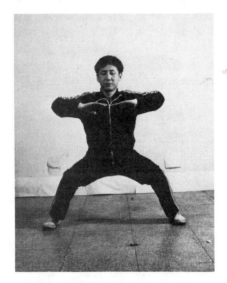

Figure 1

Left arm is stretched forward to the left, palm facing front, elbow slightly dropped and fingertips at eye level. The right hand is clenched into fist and placed near right cheek, palm facing inward. Keep right armpit hollow. Look at tip of left middle finger.

3. Embrace Tree Trunk Posture of the Shaolin School (Fig. 3)

Stand firmly with feet parallel to each other and shoulder-width apart, knees slightly bent

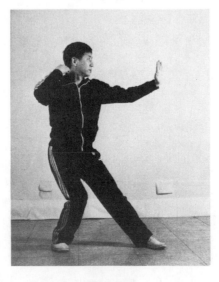

Figure 2

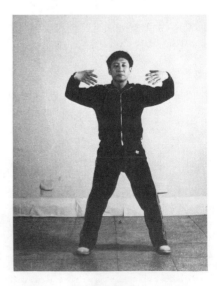

Figure 3

and trunk held upright. Curve both arms at shoulder level with elbows slightly dropped, as if you were trying to get your arms around the trunk of a big tree.

All fingers are spread out and slightly curved as if you were holding a big ball. Look straight ahead with half-closed eyes.

4. Clasp-horse posture of the Taiji School (Fig. 4)

Stand firmly with feet turned inward and knees brought close to each other. The whole posture is a bit lower than the preceding one. Other points are more or less the same.

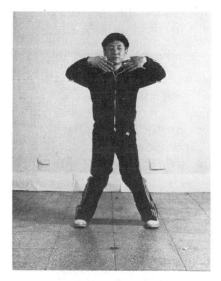

Figure 4

5. Three-in-one posture of the Xingyi (Form-and-Will) School (Fig. 5)

Same as the on guard posture of the Shaolin School except that left arm is stretched forward to the left, with elbow slightly bent, palm hollowed and facing obliquely downward, fingers separated, and the tip of middle finger at eye level.

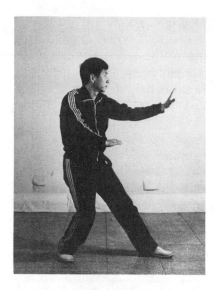

Figure 5

The right hand is placed in front of abdomen, with the root knuckle of thumb touching navel. Keep thumbs separated from fingers as far as possible. Look at the index finger of left hand.

6. Keep-good-health posture of the Xingyi School (Fig. 6)

Stand firmly as you do in the "embrace tree trunk" posture, with palms either facing inward as if you were holding something, or facing outward as if you were pushing something out.

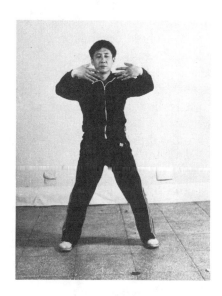

Figure 6

Hands may be placed anywhere between eye and navel levels and not farther than 30 cm from the body. Other points are the same as those for the "embrace tree trunk" posture.

7. On Guard posture of the Xingyi School (Fig. 7)

Stand firmly with left foot in front, about 60 cm away from right foot, which bears 70 percent of body weight. Both feet are turned outward. The toes of left foot press the ground and the left knee pushes forward. Draw in hips and move torso backward and downward as if to take a seat.

Separate arms, with left palm in front and both palms facing outward and positioned between eye and shoulder level, as if you were pushing something away. Other points are the same as those for the On Guard posture of the Shaolin School.

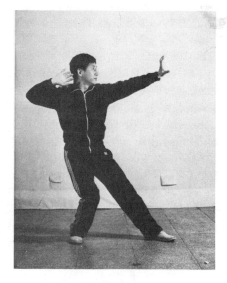

Figure 7

8. Ride-horse posture of the Southern School (Fig. 8)

Stand firmly in a half squat with feet about 45 cm apart and knees in a vertical line with toe

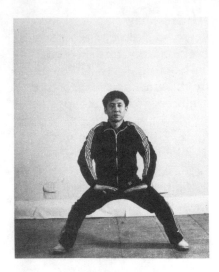

Figure 8

tips. Hands are placed in front of abdomen with palms facing down, elbows slightly bent, wrists lightly dropped and middle fingers pointing at each other. Other points are the same as those for the Ride-horse posture of the Shaolin School.

You may choose one or two postures for practice as you like. Pay attention to the following points:

1. Relax yourself from head, neck and shoulders down to arms and hands, and from chest, back, abdomen, waist, and hips down to legs and feet. Cast away all distracting thoughts and keep a tranquil mood. Relaxing before taking standing exercises is the key to success.

When practicing, think of the dantian acupuncture point. Breathe naturally. As time goes on, you will form the habit of abdominal breathing, which will produce a strong massaging effect on the stomach and intestines, and thus help improve digestive function.

Then you may start the practice of "conscious breathing," in which you imagine to yourself that the inhaled air "sinks" from the nose to the dantian and, after a little pause, comes out through the same passage. Breathing must be deep, even and slow.

2. Learn to take each posture correctly at the very beginning, with the whole body relaxed. Practice with a high degree of concentration of mind and a natural expression on the face. Keep head and trunk erect, chest and chin drawn in, mouth gently closed and tip of tongue touching upper tooth ridge. Do not protrude buttocks or raise shoulders.

3. Don't do any reading or vigorous exercise before practicing. Do not wear too much clothing. Loosen your collar and belt, and relieve yourself, if necessary. Always be in a cheerful mood.

4. Control the amount of exercise properly. For a beginner, half an hour will do for each workout. Aches in waist, legs, or knees are quite normal at the initial stage of training, and will gradually disappear as time goes on.

Rest for a little while when you find your leg muscles quivering. Some people are over anxious for quick results and start with too low a position to be able to hold on for long, and, as a result of over exertion, they may even experience palpitation, gasping, and a feeling of suffocation in the chest.

To avoid these ill effects, the standing position should be lowered stage by stage until you can comfortably hold your thighs parallel to the ground.

5. At the end of a session, cool down by massaging muscles, limbering up knee joints, and swinging legs in order to remove fatigue.

6. Exercise in a quiet place where the air is fresh, preferably after getting up or before going to bed. Do not practice within one-and-a-half hours of a meal.

Experience shows that regular practice of the standing exercise will bring about the following results:

A. It will increase your leg power, springing ability, and the gripping power of toes, which are necessary for maintaining firm stances and correct postures in all wushu routines.

B. It will help enhance the muscular strength of arms, back, and hips as well as the flexibility of joints.

C. By concentrating your thoughts on the dantian, it will help strengthen the protective inhibition of your cerebral cortex, so that your cerebrum can have ample rest. That is why you will feel relaxed, cheerful, and clear-minded after the exercise. In addition, the breathing movement during the practice will help not only to increase your vital capacity, but also improve the functions of your internal organs.

All this will, to varying degrees, contribute to curing certain chronic diseases, such as heart troubles, hypertension, neurasthenia, tracheitis, hepatitis, rheumarthritis, and gastrointestinal ailments.

PART III

BENEFITS OF QIGONG PRACTICE

By LI BAOQI

Reporter, China Sports Magazine

Qigong is a most valuable part of China's medical legacy. Originally used only for keeping fit, it was later adopted also as a curative means and has proved its worth in both respects through long years of practice.

The wonderful effects of qigong have yet to be fully explained in the light of modern science. Initial studies have amply shown how with correct ways of breathing, qigong helps to regulate the equilibrium in the higher nervous system and other systems of the human body.

It also helps promote the normal functions of different organs and build up inner strength — all conducive to stronger resistance to diseases and to better health.

So far as the nervous system is concerned, qigong helps to regulate the equilibrium between excitation and inhibition. For those who suffer from neurasthenia, practicing qigong will make them feel relaxed and gradually improve their sleep. With respect to the respiratory system, qigong can improve the function of the lungs and increase vital capacity.

While the average person normally breathes 17 or 18 times per minute, one who persists in qigong practice can breathe two or three times a minute during exercise without feeling out of breath.

Circulation and Blood Pressure Improved

Qigong aids blood circulation for the benefit of the heart. Different kinds of qigong methods can be used to adjust blood pressure. Supplemented by other therapeutic methods, they can cure diseases such as high blood pressure and arteriosclerosis.

Qigong exercises also produce obvious effects on the digestive system. Among other things, they promote digestion by stimulating the gastrointestinal movements and the secretion of digestive juice. That's why those who regularly practice qigong usually have a good appetite and seldom suffer from constipation.

Qigong hastens metabolism in the human body, activates secretion in various glands, and helps to keep one's body weight at a normal level. It also helps to stabilize one's frame of mind.

There are many kinds of qigong exercises. They may be classified according to body postures, such as lying, sitting, and standing. One who has a weak constitution should start with the lying posture and gradually progress to exercises in the sitting and standing positions as he grows stronger. Never try the three postures all at the same time.

Points to remember during qigong practice:

1. Breathe naturally, softly and rhythmically, and do not draw out your breath with force.

2. No matter which posture you may adopt, position yourself in a way that you can feel your whole body is comfortably relaxed.

3. Try to integrate movement and stillness in your exercise program. Generally speaking, taijiquan is a kind of moving exercise in qigong. So, besides doing static qigong exercises, it will do you good to practice a little taijiquan or some other active forms of fitness exercises.

4. Be patient and persevere when you practice qigong and do not seek immediate results.

Although qigong can be used to keep fit and cure disease, it is no panacea. Good results can be achieved only when we combine it with other methods of physical training and medical treatment in a way that best suits the conditions of each individual.

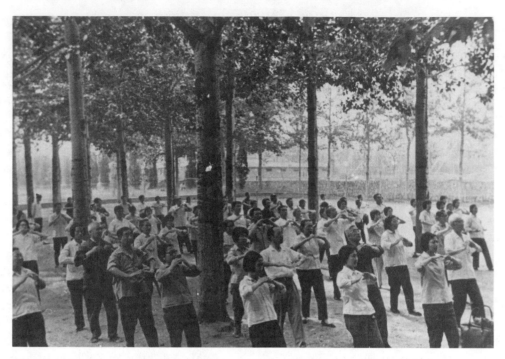

Thousands upon thousands of people have benefited from qigong practice.

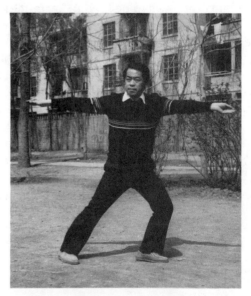

Fan Zeng, a famous painter, practicing the popular Flying Crane exercise.

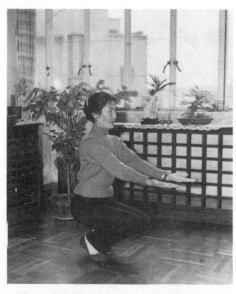

Qigong exercises help to keep Zhang Ruifang, a well-known film actress, in good health.

MA CHUN — A QIGONG MASTER

By HU BAOYAN

Teacher at Beihong Middle School, Shanghai

Qigong is known to have worked wonders. A splendid heritage of Chinese culture, it serves as a means of keeping fit and helps cure chronic diseases and prolong one's life. Now a new aspect of its virtues — curing certain cancers — is being explored and studied by some qigong practitioners and research workers. One of the pioneers in this field is Ma Chun, deputy director of the Institute of Traditional Chinese Medicine, Shanghai. The story of his achievements has been published in *The New York Times*.

Ma Chun was brought up in Majiazhuang (Ma Family Village), Shandong Province, where qigong and wushu had thrived. As legend has it, they were brought there by five monks who had fled from the Shaolin Monastery of Shandong Province — a branch of the renowned Shaolin Monastery of Songshan in Henan — to escape a bloody suppression by emperor Yong Zheng of the Qing Dynasty (1644-1911), who feared that the monks of the temple might assassinate him.

Ma started to practice wushu at seven and distinguished himself for his strength and skill. At 14, he joined the Eighth Route Army during the War of Resistance Against Japan (1937-45) and was a scout and later captain of an armed detachment in the enemy-occupied area. During the War of Liberation (1946-49), he was promoted to be the commander of the guards' company under Marshal Chen Yi (1901-1972).

During intervals between battles, he seized every opportunity to practice wushu exercises which strengthened his body and enabled him to acquit himself of various duties splendidly. Once when he was chased by a group of enemy soldiers who were closing in on him, he leaped over a sorghum stalk fence higher than his own body, thereby shaking off his pursuers.

He had a pair of sharp eyes able to see objects thousands of meters away, the result of constantly exercising his eyes since childhood. He was once wounded in the back. He did not go to a doctor or use any medicine, but he gradually recovered with the aid of qigong.

After the liberation in 1949, Ma Chun continued his training of qigong under the guidance of an old monk in the Wutai Mountain. Incorporating what he had learned with what he had inherited from his ancestors, he developed a school of his own.

Amazing Effects of Qigong

Qigong has the special effect of regulating the disorders of the internal organs and nerves, facilitating blood circulation and, therefore, helping reduce swellings and eliminating nodes. Over the years, Ma Chun has been quite successful in using qigong to treat common diseases like hypertension, cardiovascular and gastroenteric disorders, bronchial asthma, neurasthenia, and gynaecological diseases.

About 90 percent of a group of hypertension sufferers who learned the art from him had their blood pressure lowered after just a month's practice. Their conditions practically returned to normal within three months. Some patients of serious neurasthenia often found themselves in a state of trance and their faces looked yellowish pale. After taking up qigong exercises, they not only slept well but had rosy cheeks. Ma has devised a special set of exercises called the "Red-crest Crane Steps," which help limber up the limbs and fingers as well as the body.

The movements of bending up and down in coordination with relaxed breathing achieve the purpose of massaging the internal organs and, therefore, are particularly efficacious to curing diseases of the digestive system.

Assimilating the essentials of the Darmor School of qigong, he has evolved a series of standing exercises which include the leopard, tiger, crane, dragon, and snake styles of boxing, each of which has special effects on certain areas of the body. They are all especially good for juniors. The leopard style of boxing, for instance, is to increase physical power and the tiger style of boxing strengthens the bones.

In 1980, Ma Chun was invited to give a demonstration of his school of qigong on TV in Beijing and Zhejiang Province. After the demonstration he was snowed under with letters of praise from viewers who said that his exercises were simple, easy to learn, and effective in curing chronic disease.

For the benefit of those eager to learn, the Institute of Traditional Chinese Medicine in Shanghai held a qigong class directed by Ma Chun himself. Of the 148 people who suffered from various kinds of chronic diseases, 27 recovered or greatly improved their health after two months of practice and 81 showed signs of gradual recovery. The exercises were particularly effective for the digestive and locomotor systems.

"Magic Palms"

Through constant practice, Ma Chun is able to exude through his fingers or palms a kind of energy called "waiqi" (or outflowing energy) which he discovered by chance in 1967 could cure certain diseases. He began to frequent a tumor hospital and tried his brand-new "weapon" on the patients.

To his amazement, his waiqi succeeded where both Western and Chinese medicines had failed. The patients' pains were alleviated and their "incurable disease" was cured. The news that Dr. Ma had a pair of "magic palms" soon spread among patients suffering from cancer.

Waving or pushing his palms from a distance of about one foot at the patient's diseased part, Ma Chun emits his waiqi from the "laogongxue," an acupuncture point on his hand. Immediately the patient feels a kind of current coursing through his body, a feeling of numbness, cold and heat similar to that caused by a needle inserted into an acupuncture point on the patient's body.

One of the patients Ma Chun cured had suffered from compression fracture of the lumbar vertebrae and had been confined to his bed in a hospital for a long time. When Ma Chun released his waiqi at his waist from a distance of 40 cm, the patient felt a current of heat throughout his body. There was sweat on the tip of his nose and a rhythmic beat in some parts of his muscles. After only 20 days of treatment, he was cured and left the hospital.

Another patient was a middle-aged woman who had contracted uterus tumor. After Ma Chun gave her treatment, her conditions gradually improved. She learned qigong from Ma and, through persistent exercise, her tumor which had grown to the size of a fist simply disappeared.

Waiqi Identified

In recent years, research work has been conducted to determine the nature of the invisible and intangible waiqi, and it has now been identified as a kind of modulated infrared radiation having the characteristics of magnetics, electricity, light waves, micro-particle currents, neutrons, beta rays and supersonics.

Clinical experiments have also revealed that waiqi, which is a highly centralized energy, not only can kill certain cancer cells which are later discharged from the body but also raise the degree of immunity from such diseases. Though its therapeutic effect has been ascertained in treating cancer of the thyroid gland, esophagus, stomach, and rectum, much still remains to be explored.

Good-natured and composed and not easily provoked to anger, 60-year-old Ma Chun is hale and hearty. His face glows with health and his gait is springy and brisk. He only sleeps two or three hours a day and goes regularly through his qigong routines from 11 p.m. to 1 a.m. In order to pass on his qigong knowledge, he has been diligently working on several books. His "Body-Building Qigong" was published in 1981 by the People's Sports Publishing House in Beijing.

Now a leading member of the Qigong Scientific Research Institute of China, he often gives free treatment to the sick during his spare hours.

"China is the home of qigong, I'm duty bound to help develop this traditional art and at the same time do my bit to serve the people." These words well illustrate Ma Chun's lofty aspirations and dedication to improving the people's health.

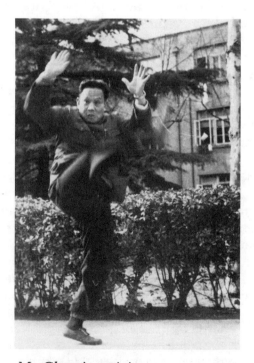

Ma Chun in training.

INDEED A DIFFERENT MAN

By HU BIN

Professor at Beijing College of Traditional Chinese Medicine

I am 70 years old. At 51 I began to suffer from a number of chronic diseases — neurasthenia, high blood pressure, cerebral arteriosclerosis, coronary disease and hepatosplenomegaly (coincident liver and spleen enlargement). I was treated with both Chinese and Western medicine, but to no avail. I became too weak to carry on my work.

It was a case of either overcoming these diseases or being overcome by them. It occurred to me that perhaps I had done too much mental work and too little physical exercise over the years, which had led to functional disorders of my central and autonomic nervous systems, and that I might try readjusting these through qigong and other exercises along with medication. So I planned for myself a regimen consisting of three treatment phases, each lasting three months.

In the first phase, medication was primary and qigong exercises secondary. I took various kinds of medicines, first of all to stop angina pectoris, and then gradually to invigorate the functions of my heart and brain and to lower my cholesterol level.

At the same time I began to do qigong exercises four times a day. By the end of the third month, I had become better both physically and mentally. Such symptoms as dizziness, headache, shortness of breath, palpitation and pain in the chest had been markedly alleviated. My blood pressure had returned to near normal. Angina pectoris had stopped. Insomnia had become less of a problem. Whenever I couldn't get to sleep I would sit up and practice qigong in bed.

Insomnia and Blood Pressure Controlled

In the second stage, qigong exercises became primary and medication secondary. The result was that in addition to the disappearance of the symptoms mentioned above, constipation and rectal spasms ceased. In time, my insomnia and high blood pressure, which had plagued me for 10 years, were brought under control without the use of pills. Hemihyperhidrosis (localized excessive sweating) and numbness of the body and limbs rarely occurred, except when I was overtired.

In the third phase, stress was laid on physical training to consolidate the benefits already obtained. With a better appetite, I was gaining weight and strength. After each qigong exercise period I was in good spirits — energetic, cheerful, relaxed and at ease. I was now ready to work part time.

In the 19 years since then, my coronary disease and cerebral arteriosclerosis have been kept in check, and my neurasthenia, high blood pressure and hepatosplenomegaly have radically improved. The secret of it all lies in persistent practice of qigong and other exercises, which help in mobilizing the potential energy in the human body and enhancing its ability to resist and overcome diseases.

Ancient Chinese hygienists maintained that the human body was made up of three essentials, namely, "yi" (mind), "qi" (energy) and "jing" (hormones), and that one would live to a robust old age by nursing these essentials but would die young if one dissipated them. Qigong exercises are precisely meant for the preservation of these essentials.

Through the exercise of "yi" one regulates his mental condition and enjoys a state of tranquility. Through the exercise of qi one expands his vital capacity and promotes blood circulation. Through the exercise of "jing" one readjusts the body's internal balance and builds up physical vitality.

Today, at 70, I have a good memory, a strong heart, a sound body and a ruddy face, which, were it not for the thin grey hair on my head, would well belie my age. Indeed, I am now quite different from what I was 19 years ago — thanks to the life-giving effects of qigong.

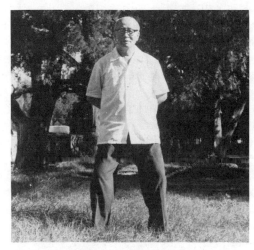

Seventy-year-old Hu Bin doing a qigong exercise.

A WOMAN WHO SAVED
HER OWN AND MANY OTHER LIVES

By GAO YUN

Editor, People's Sports Publishing House, Beijing

Moving about on the velvety grass — now like a crane flapping its wings, now like a tiger prancing on a prey, now like a monkey toying with a newly plucked peach . . . she is actually doing a set of fitness exercises called "Five-Animal Play," which may be traced back to the third century A.D. Looking at her nimble movements, one would hardly believe that she is 73 and still less that she once suffered from a number of diseases — tuberculosis, arthritis, heart troubles, and, last but not least, cancer.

A Life-and-Death Struggle

This old lady, Professor Guo Lin, has, for nearly half of her lifetime, been engaged in a grim struggle with death. And she owes her triumph to qigong, an ancient Chinese form of keep-fit exercise characterized by full activation of qi.

Guo Lin was born in Guangdong's Zhongshan County — the birthplace of Dr. Sun Yat-sen, under whose leadership her father devoted his life to the Revolution of 1911, which ended the monarchy of the Qing Dynasty.

Orphaned at age two, Guo Lin lived with her grandfather, who was a famous qigong master and taught her the basics of the art. Guo was found with cancer in the uterus at age 40. The tumor spread to other parts of her body and she had to go through six operations in eight years, leaving her completely enfeebled.

But she did not abandon herself to despair. She recalled the qigong exercises and five-animal play she had learned in childhood. But she soon found that they ill suited her health condition, which was going from bad to worse. Whenever she tried to concentrate and go into meditation, the thought of imminent death would haunt her. Being too weak to summon up her vital energy, she would doze off in the midst of a sitting.

It occurred to her that she might work out a new routine for her own use. So she delved into a comparative study of the conventional schools of qigong and devised a set of "walking exercises" that combined meditation with movements. It proved most refreshing when she performed it at dawn in the park.

Summarizing her intensive studies of qigong theories and her own therapeutic experience, Guo Lin has written a book entitled, "Qigong: A New Method for Combating Cancer." It is the first treatise ever written in China on this subject. Starting from 1973, she has given many lectures on qigong therapy and conducted four courses: primary, secondary and advanced classes for ordinary chronic diseases and one for cancer.

The exercises she teaches fall into three main categories:

1. Natural Walking Exercises: These involve slow steps and arm swings coordinated with breathing.

2. Stick-rolling Exercises: The patient holds a 30 cm-long stick in his hands, rolling it gently between his palms while squatting and turning his trunk to right and left. The movements are synchronized with respiration.

3. Utterance Exercises: The patient utters long-drawn-out sounds, such as "ah," "yi," and "hi," according to different parts of the body affected by tumor.

During the past decade or so, Guo's qigong exercises have cured tens of thousands of chronically ill patients. Available case histories show that some 300 cancer patients have achieved notable results by practicing these exercises. Here are two typical examples:

Yu Dayuan, a member of the army's song and dance troupe, was already in the advanced stage of rectum cancer when he entered Guo's therapy class in 1977. The daily qigong practice has greatly sharpened his appetite and improved his health. In spite of the trouble caused by the changed course of his anus after an early operation, he is working half day on his regular job. In addition, he spends one hour every morning teaching a qigong class as a voluntary instructor.

Li Shurong, a 41-year-old worker at the "February 7" Rolling Stock Plant, got breast cancer in 1973. After the incision of her right breast, new tumors were discovered in the left breast, leading to many complications and a nervous breakdown.

Then she turned to Guo Lin, not without misgivings. But her doubts began to vanish when she found that she could sleep better and eat more. By the end of the first six months in the qigong class, the syndrome had disappeared and she happily returned to her job in 1978. She has now survived as many as seven years.

Although numerous facts have proved the benefits of qigong exercises in curing chronic diseases, cancer included, no satisfactory answer has been given to explain the way it works. From the viewpoint of traditional Chinese medicine, it is presumed that by doing Guo's walking exercises which combine physical and mental activities through movement, meditation and regulated breathing, a patient can summon up his internal vital energy.

This brings about a balance between the positive and negative elements in his body, clears his internal organs of obstructions and promotes circulation in his blood vessels, thereby aiding his recovery.

Initial investigations indicate that those cancer patients who do the walking qigong exercises regularly develop a greater ability in their phagocytes to destroy cancer cells. At the same time, they find it easier to withstand the side-effects of radiation and chemotherapies.

An Artist as Well

Guo Lin is also a famous artist versed in traditional Chinese painting. She founded an academy at age 30 and has since trained hundreds of painters. The Chinese Fine Artists' Association has sponsored two exhibitions of her works, which are highly appreciated for her unique style and expressive power in depicting landscapes with the brush and Chinese ink.

"I took up painting by accident," Guo told me with great gusto in my interview with her. "I was a tomboy, so to speak, in my school days, for I always wore a man's suit and had my hair cut short. I even won a gold medal in a 10,000-meter race!

"My teacher of fine arts despised me for my stubbornness and lack of femininity and gave me 59.9 for my exam — just 0.1 below the passing mark. So I made up my mind to surpass him. Life is full of adversities which may sometimes be turned to good account. But for that humiliating mark, I wouldn't have become an artist; but for cancer, I wouldn't have become a master of qigong, would I?"

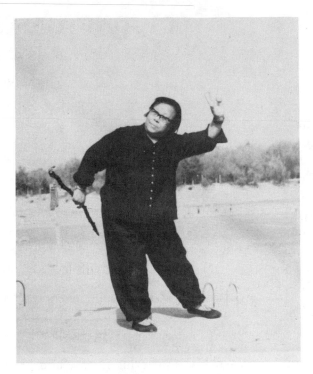

Guo Lin practicing her own version of the 'Five-Animal Play.'

QIGONG HAS WORKED WONDERS

By ZHOU SHIYUAN

Staff Member, Qinghua University, Beijing

Sometimes people make acquaintances in unusual circumstances, and many of mine were made, of all places in the world, at a qigong coaching center, where we were thrown together by the common misfortune of ill health. But later we also shared the good fortune of becoming fit again.

Our coaching center, one of the hundreds in Beijing, is run by the teachers' union of Qinghua University, a polytechnic institute founded in 1911, which now has 18 departments and a total enrollment of some 10,000.

After my graduation from Qinghua's department of hydraulic engineering in 1970, I stayed at the university as a researcher. But during the first decade of my career I was on sick leave for more than four years. I was suffering from a number of ailments — neurasthenia, gastroenteritis, hepatitis and arthritis, to mention but a few.

I was hospitalized for a couple of years and went through three operations, which left me pining away in debility and despaired of life.

One day in the spring of 1980, a friend of mine told me that a qigong coaching center was going to be set up on our campus, with the famous qigong master Guo Lin as the head instructor. "Why don't you join it?" he said. "Many people with chronic diseases have recovered by doing Professor Guo's exercises. Maybe they'll do you some good."

Qigong Saved His Life

Though doubting whether qigong would be effective in my case, I decided to try it — just to try. A drowning man will catch at a straw, won't he? And, as it turned out, this straw of qigong really saved my life!

Our qigong course covered a period of three months, with a two-hour workout every week. After learning some movements, we were required to practice them by ourselves, at least for half an hour every day.

The training load was quite heavy for those in delicate health. With seven-tenths of my stomach cut off, my bowels always running loose and my knees plagued with constant pain, I could hardly stick out a training session at the beginning, even though the exercises were very slow and light. After doing them for a few minutes, I would be out of breath and sweat profusely.

Several times I thought of calling it quits. But I banished the idea when I recalled my instructor's words: "Perseverance means victory. Sweetness will come after bitterness."

Sure enough, hardly had a month passed when my bowel movement began to improve. Seeing a ray of hope, I kept on doing the exercises with increased confidence. A few months later I began to have a good appetite.

In October of that year, I was strong enough to work four hours a day. Two years later, I resumed full time work and, in addition, gave two lectures a week at an evening school. Now my regular job is the publication of a newsletter for the alumni of Qinghua University and I spend the evenings writing articles for some journals.

Sometimes I spend my leisure hours with my chorus group, which gives performances now and then on festive occasions. Of course, I never pass a day without doing qigong exercises, at least one hour daily.

900 of 1,000 Benefited

All my relatives and friends say that I have changed a lot these years, both physically and in mental attitude. Indeed, I've not only recovered my health, but also rediscovered the meaning of life. Nothing brings me greater joy than the knowledge that I can render useful service to society.

And I'm glad that many others have had the same experience. Among the 1,000 patients graduated from the qigong coaching center, 900 have benefited from the exercises to a greater or lesser extent. Here are just a few examples:

Chen Lizhen, lecturer at the chemical engineering department, was found in 1979 to have contracted cancer in her oral cavity. After an operation, the doctors suggested radiation treatment — either over a large area which might save her life but at the expense of her eyesight, or over a small area which would save her eyesight but at the risk of her very life.

After much agonizing hesitation, she chose the latter course, thinking that she might take up qigong exercises as a supplementary measure to radiotherapy. She entered our qigong center in 1980 and has survived to this day, active in work and full of confidence.

Sun Shagong, a mechanic at one of our experimental workshops, had suffered for a dozen years from a blood tumor as big as an egg in his lower back, which forced him to lie on his belly night after night. Since he took up qigong exercises in 1980, the tumor has gradually disappeared. He often shows the old affected part to others, saying elatedly, "Just feel it. That devil's given me the slip!"

Can Jianyi, a clerk at the computer department, had suffered from hepatitis and stayed in a hospital for more than three years before 1980. His relatives were already preparing for his funeral. As the last resort, he struggled out of his sick bed and staggered to the training ground of our qigong center. Now he is in normal shape and he even took part in the cross-country and 800 meter races at the last two intramural athletic meets.

In citing these examples, I don't mean that qigong is a panacea. The treatment of chronic diseases is after all a highly complicated problem and involves many factors. Yet there is no denying the fact that qigong exercises can help, in one way or another, to improve the functions of various organs and systems in the human body. This is of vital importance to our fight against illness.

In practicing qigong exercises, a patient should coordinate them with other curative measures, such as medication, chemotherapy or radiotherapy. Besides, he should keep a cheerful mood, for mental health always plays an important role in practicing qigong and treating chronic diseases.

Some people have achieved little or no effect in doing qigong exercises because they go about it by fits and starts or give up midway. Good results will not come overnight, nor even in a fortnight. Carry on for months and years — under correct guidance, of course — and qigong will do much good to your health and work wonders in curing your illness.

It is precisely owing to its long-tested therapeutic value that qigong has been handed down from generation to generation and is now practiced by millions of people in China.

I'm glad that plans are underway to carry out theoretical studies of qigong by utilizing our university's laboratories and research personnel and the rich experience accumulated by our coaching center. Undoubtedly this will give impetus to the advancement of qigong as a branch of life science.

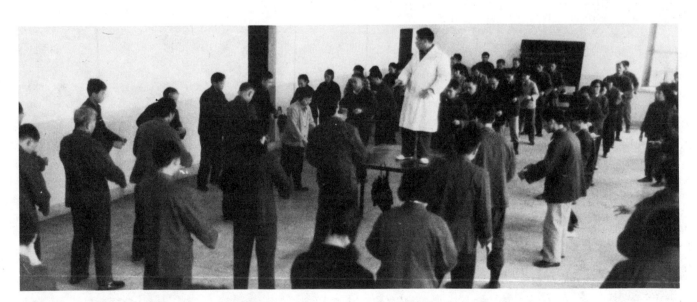

A qigong class for patients of chronic diseases conducted by Wang Xinde, a practitioner at the Research Society of Traditional Chinese Medicine, Zhejiang Province.

KURIMOTO IS CURED OF HIS BACKACHE

By GAO YUN

Editor, People's Sports Publishing House, Beijing

One day in May 1981, a Japanese guest made a call on Liang Lizhen, formerly a world-famous table tennis player and now a deputy director of the Physical Culture and Sports Commission of Guangdong Province. He was Mr. Kurimoto Takaro, who had come to China to attend the Guangzhou Spring Trade Fair. His wife, Kumijo Matsuzaki, twice world table tennis champion, has been a good friend of Liang's since the early 1960s.

Liang was not a little surprised to see her guest in a stiff posture. He told her that he had been plagued with backache for five years. It had recurred shortly before he left Japan, so that he had to board the plane with the help of his wife. The pain had worsened after he arrived in Guangzhou, obviously as a result of his busy work at the fair.

"Why not try the traditional Chinese medical treatment?" Liang suggested. "I know some doctors here who are specialized in qigong and acupuncture. They've cured lots of patients like you."

The treatment took place in a quiet corner of a park. Kurimoto was asked to sit relaxedly on a rock. After doing a breathing exercise, a qigong master named Liang Qifeng concentrated his qi in his right palm, which he moved up and down behind Kurimoto's back.

The qi current emanated like X-rays to penetrate the affected part of the body. Instantly, the patient felt a tingling yet soothing sensation in his lower back. Then he was massaged on the shoulders. Finally much of his pain was gone, and he could bend forward to touch his knees with his hands.

Two days later, Kurimoto had an engagement with another doctor, Zhu Gaozhang — this time for an acupuncture treatment. Turning up the patient's upper lip, Dr. Zhu found a tiny white spot on the gum. He pricked it with a needle to let out a little blood. Kurimoto wondered: What has my gum to do with my back? But all his doubts vanished when he stood up and found he could bend forward and touch the floor. "Wonderful, very wonderful!" he cried out with joy. "I'm as light as a bird."

Kurimoto's quick recovery soon became the talk of the hotel. There was a phone call from his anxious wife that evening. Kurimoto told her everything.

"Tell my friend Liang Lizhen," said an excited voice at the other end of the line, "I'll always remember her. I'll always remember those wonderful doctors!"

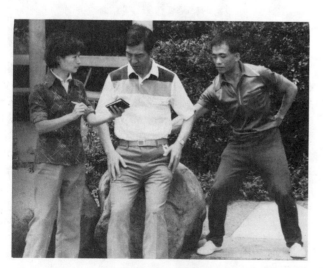

Kurimoto receives qigong treatment from Liang Qifeng, a master of the art.

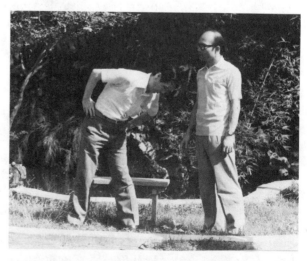

Kurimoto can move about freely after acupuncture treatment by Dr. Zhu Gaozhang.

QIGONG IN THE FIGHT AGAINST CANCER

By GE XIAN

Reporter, People's Daily

One evening last spring, I paid a visit to Gao Wenbin, a 59-year-old Navy officer who had contracted cancer of the lung four years ago. As he showed me into his living room, I noticed that his gait was steady and his face glowed with health. He certainly looked much better than he did the last time I met him two years ago.

Then a group of cancer patients were practicing qigong one early morning in a little wood in the Longtan Lake Park in Beijing. On a nearby stone bench sat Gao, his face pale with weakness. He told me that he had improved somewhat after more than a year's qigong practice. But, he remarked, "time will show how effective it is."

And now, two years later, I was pleasantly surprised to find him in good health.

"I used to be rather weak, but qigong has made me stronger."

After pouring out a cup of tea for me, my host went on talking with animation.

"I get up after three in the morning and start practicing qigong at about four. Every day I spend a few hours doing the exercises before going to office."

"Do you go to work regularly?" I was a bit curious.

"Why, yes! And besides, from time to time I receive urgent calls that keep me busy in the evening."

As if to confirm his words, the telephone on his desk rang.

After receiving the phone call, Gao told me his story in detail.

Pulmonary Adenoma

"My case was diagnosed as pulmonary adenoma as early as July 1976. You know, they told me at first that it was benign, but I doubted that before long. The doctor, for instance, always tried to cover up with one hand the case history he was writing after he had given me a check-up. Why did he have to do that? I was full of misgivings.

"Two months later I happened to have the chance of looking at my case history and came to know I had cancer which had developed to a far stage. Strange to say, I felt quite at ease when I knew the truth. I would die if the worst comes to the worst, but what did that matter to a man like me who had the good fortune to survive the revolutionary wars? What I was most concerned about at that time was my work. I told myself I had to overcome the disease so that I could work for a few more years."

After taking a sip of tea, Gao continued: "It was already too late to have my lung removed. So I underwent radiotherapy and at the same time took traditional Chinese medicine to reduce the side effects. In the course of chemotherapy that followed, I felt so bad I could only eat one liang (50 grams) of cooked rice or steamed bread a meal, and I only had four or five hours of intermittent sleep every night. GPT level was high and I suffered from headache, dizziness and swollen legs. Leukocyte count dropped to 3,000."

"What made you think of taking up qigong?" I asked.

"My friends and relatives showed great concern for me," Gao replied. "One of my colleagues told me that qigong had good effects on certain diseases. Seeing my doubts, she showed me a pile of case histories she had borrowed from Guo Lin, a well-known artist of the Beijing Art Academy who had been practicing and coaching qigong exercises for decades. Many cancer patients had learned these exercises from Guo and benefited from them. So I decided to try."

No Other Way Out

On the morning of May 8, 1977, Gao went to the qigong center in the Longtan Lake Park for the first time. On meeting Guo Lin, he said, "I've come to you because I have no other way out. But I promise to be a good pupil."

And so, with what he learned from Guo Lin he began his stubborn struggle against cancer. At first he was so weak that after taking 200 "steps" for the day's exercise he could hardly lift his legs and had to clamber up his bed at night. But he went on practicing day after day and month after month, gradually increasing the number of "steps" to 10,000.

"Now I can easily do more than ten thousand steps every day," he said with a note of triumph.

"That means seven thousand meters, doesn't it?" I inquired.

"Not quite, because the steps are shorter than normal strides. But they are quick and coordinated with accelerated respiration so that the amount of exercise involved is much bigger than in walking."

Gao then went on to describe the results of the qigong exercises.

"I began to sleep well two weeks after taking up the exercises. Three or four months later, my appetite had improved so much I could eat three or four liang of cooked rice or steamed bread each meal. Symptoms of pneumonia caused by radiation had gone. My legs were no longer swollen, and my liver functions and blood picture had returned to normal.

I used to catch cold pretty often. But I am much stronger now. Wind or snow, I take qigong exercises in the open air every day, and, as far as I remember, I caught cold only once in the past three years.

"The doctor referred to my progress as a 'marvel' in the first year, a 'real marvel' in the second, and a 'miracle' in the third. And now I am in the fourth year . . . " Gao's eyes sparkled as he spoke.

Qigong Helps Prolong Life

He would have gone on talking had I not been reminded by my watch that it was time for me to take my leave. When he saw me to the door, he said, "Qigong helps to prolong the life of cancer patients. It is really worth studying."

A few days later I called on Dr. Kang Liyuan, vice-director of the Chest Surgery Department at the General Hospital of the People's Liberation Army, who had given Gao medical treatment.

On learning my purpose in coming, Dr. Kang immediately sent for Gao's case history. Then he made the following summary:

"Gao's case was identified as pulmonary adenoma by bronchoscopic visualization and biopsy in July 1976. An operation in our hospital on August 31 revealed wide dissemination of cancer cells to the lymph glands in the thorax mediastinum and hilus of the lung. Total removal of the lung was given up as meaningless. Radiotherapy was administered from September 16 to October 11. Chemotherapy was started on January 21, 1977. Three courses of treatment were envisaged, but in the end only one was given."

"What was the result of the treatment?" I asked.

"Gao's case was classified as belonging to the metastatic stage. Although there wasn't yet dissemination to distant parts of the body, the thorax mediastinum and hilus of the lung were already involved. His case was T1 N2 M0.

"Ordinarily, a cancer patient of that late stage can expect to survive only one year if he does not undergo any treatment, or if he does undergo treatment but shows no response to it, or if he has to stop having treatment because he can't endure it. It is really beyond our expectation that Gao Wenbin could have lived on for almost four years."

"Has this something to do with qigong?" I finally came to the point.

"Well," the doctor said, seeming to have ignored my question, "there are many ways of combating cancer. I am a surgeon, and I know surgical excision at an early stage is quite effective for lung cancer. According to figures compiled by some hospitals, 30 or 40 per cent or the patients treated this way have survived up to five years.

But surgical excision was out of the question for Gao, who could only be given radiotherapy and chemotherapy. A total dosage of 7,000 rads was administered on him, and in chemotherapy we prescribed fluorouracil deoxyribonucleoside, which should be quite effective against glandular cancers. Unfortunately, it was too strong for him and we had to give up after one course of treatment.

"While radiation and chemotherapy are undeniably important means of treatment, they have a number of side effects. First, they take away the patient's appetite; second, they may cause radiation pneumonia; and third, they reduce the number of blood platelets and leukocyte count and weaken the patient, sometimes to the point of giving up treatment altogether.

Unique in Its Effects

"As for qigong, it should be regarded as yet another method of treatment, which has proved its unique effects in enhancing appetite, restoring physical strength and building up health.

"By the way, have you visited Dr. Yu Rencun, director of the Tumours Department at the Beijing Hospital of Traditional Chinese Medicine? Gao Wenbin has been taking Chinese medicine prescribed by him."

Director Yu, as I learned afterwards, was at first a doctor of the Western school but later took up the study and practice of Chinese medicine. Recalling his experience with Gao Wenbin when I called on him, Dr. Yu said:

"Our prognosis for him was very unfavorable and it really surprised us that he could have lived for such a long time. Since surgical excision was not adopted, he must have experienced pathological changes. Radiotherapy and chemotherapy destroy cancer cells, but not completely.

"Using traditional Chinese medicine to 'foster what is sound and suppress what is unhealthy,' some patients can live several years with cancer in their bodies. Gao Wenbin has been taking Chinese medicine ever since he was put under treatment, and that has reduced the side effects of radiation and chemotherapy.

His condition further improved after he took up qigong exercises, which like Chinese medicine help to regulate the function of vital energy and the state of the blood, maintain the equilibrium of internal environments and strengthen the natural defenses of the body against cancer."

As he spoke, he took a classical book from his shelf and showed me a passage in it.

"This was written in the Ming Dynasty several hundred years ago," he explained. "It described how daoyin, a form of qigong exercise, was applied in curing cancer of the esophagus."

As I jotted down some notes from the book, I thought to myself, "So the use of qigong in curing cancer is not a fancy idea. It is a time-honored method that dates back several centuries."

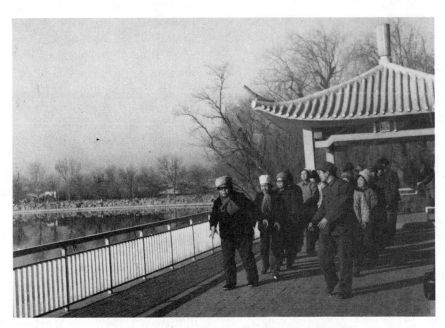

Guo Lin leading a group of patients in qigong exercise.

QIGONG BENEFITS CANCER PATIENTS

By CAI ZENG

Reporter, Sports News

In or near every park in Beijing, you'll find many people, separately or in groups, doing qigong exercises. Some are walking with slow, big strides or swinging their arms and some are standing still in "ride-horse" posture like a Buddha in meditation.

In the long course of its development, qigong was tinged with mysticism and regarded as superstition and trickery.

It is only in recent years that this ancient art has regained its reputation and attracted increasing interest among medical personnel and patients of cancer and chronic diseases.

Since the establishment of the Beijing Qigong Institute in December 1979, about a dozen coaching stations have been set up in parks and even more in factories and government organs. There are now some 300 instructors teaching thousands of patients how to do qigong exercises for preventive and curative purposes.

According to a study made by the Beijing Qigong Institute, out of a total of 3,100 patients of chronic diseases who have practiced qigong for 3-5 years, 25 percent have recovered completely, 44 percent have improved remarkably and 22 percent satisfactorily. The remaining 9 percent have made no progress.

I interviewed some cancer patients at the coaching stations in three parks — the Purple Bamboo Park, the Labouring People's Cultural Palace and the Temple of Earth. Here are their stories:

Zhang Huisheng, 48, head nurse at the No. 1 Hospital of Beijing Medical College:

"In April 1979, I found I had got breast cancer and I underwent an operation immediately. As a nurse, I knew quite well that only 50-60 percent of breast cancer patients could survive beyond five years. I had looked after quite a few who died some time after operation.

Couldn't Believe Qigong Could Help

"Whenever I closed my eyes, their agonized faces would appear before me. Quietly and sadly I was preparing to meet my inevitable doom. One day, someone told me that qigong might help me. I couldn't believe it. But on second thought, I decided that there was no harm in trying. So I came to the Purple Bamboo Park, where I found a lot of cancer patients doing qigong exercises. Many told me that it really worked. They kindled a ray of hope in me.

"In the beginning, I was so weak that I would get tired after a few minutes exercises. But it was not long before I began to feel better and gain confidence. I've been doing qigong exercises for only a little over a year, yet they have helped me improve my health and overcome the strong side effects of the eight courses of chemotherapy I had received."

Xiao Ruinian, 41, employee at a printing house in Jingzhou City, Hubei Province:

"People say that I look in the pink of health. Who'll believe I've suffered from ovary cancer? After the diagnosis in 1973, I had two major operations and long periods of chemotherapy, which left me so weak that I would start gasping violently after taking a few steps upstairs. My abdominal muscles became stiff and I couldn't bend my trunk.

"In April last year I showed symptoms of cancer recurrence. I came to Beijing to learn qigong exercises at the coaching station run by The Cultural Palace. In a month and a half my white blood cells increased from 3,000 to 6,000 counts and the tumor shrank from 6 x 8 to 4 x 5 cm. I could eat more and sleep better and I felt stronger.

Tumor Disappears

"I returned to my native town in June and kept up with the exercises. I usually got up at 4:30 in the morning and spent three hours on the ancient city wall nearby doing exercises and singing a song or two when I felt like it. In September last year I came to Beijing again for an advanced course of qigong to consolidate the curative effect already achieved. A few days ago I had another examination. My tumor had disappeared altogether!"

Shi Zehuang, 42, doctor at the People's Hospital of Huai-an County, Jiangsu Province:

"The cancer in my pancreas was too far gone for a surgical operation when it was discovered in October 1979. My wife, also a doctor, sought the advice of many cancer specialists. They all said that my case was beyond cure. In June 1980, we read from Sports News that many cancer patients had benefited from qigong exercises.

"We also heard about the famous qigong master Guo Lin who was teaching the art in Beijing. So we packed our things and went to the capital by train. Guo said her training class was already overcrowded and she could not take any more applicants. With tears in her eyes, my wife begged again and again until Guo agreed to take me on.

"I went into the training — or rather a life-and-death struggle — in real earnest. Three months later I became a different man. I could sleep all night through and had a good appetite. I'd put on more than 10 kilos. Believe it or not, tufts of hair had reappeared on my once bald head. What made me most happy was to see my wife beaming with smiles again.

"I'm very interested in qigong, both as a doctor and a patient. We're still not very clear about the mechanism of qigong, but practice has shown that it can, according to the theory of traditional Chinese medicine, summon up one's vital energy to improve the functions of one's organs. This is very favorable for the prevention and treatment of diseases.

"Now more and more people, including myself, have realized the therapeutic value of qigong and many hospitals have adopted it as an auxiliary to medication and radiotherapy. I'm planning to use it after I return to my hospital. My own experience will certainly prove helpful."

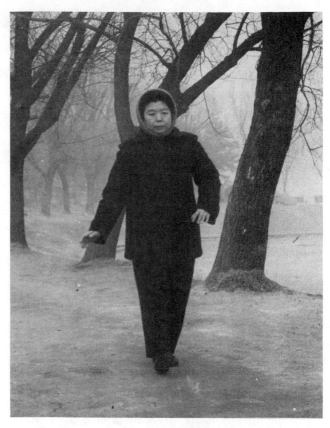

Zhang Huisheng doing qigong exercises in the Purple Bamboo Park in Beijing.

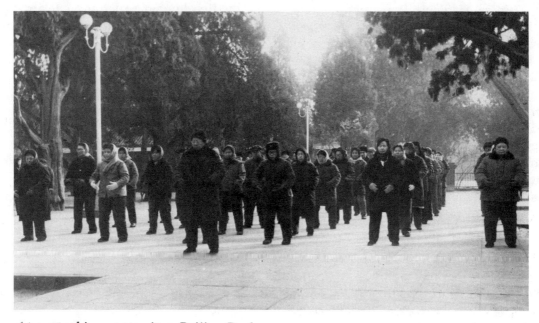

At a coaching centre in a Beijing Park.

A NEWFOUND THERAPY

By BIAN JI

Reporter, China Sports Magazine

A unique surgical operation took place on June 21, 1980, at the Shanghai No. 8 People's Hospital. A qigong master stretched out his right hand and pointed his index and middle fingers at an acupuncture point between the eyebrows of the patient.

Through his fingertips he released waiqi, or outflowing energy, from a distance of about three centimeters to anesthetize a 29-year-old woman who lay relaxed on the operation table with her eyes closed. Three minutes later, the qigong man nodded to the surgeon to start the operation for a thyroid tumor.

The patient did not show the least sign of pain. Only a casual remark betrayed her awareness of the scalpel: "How is it, doc?" Throughout the 140-minute operation, she was completely at ease, and when a nurse told her that the tumor together with the surrounding tissues the size of a walnut had been removed, a faint smile lit up her face. After the wound was stanched and sutured, she sat up slowly and nodded thanks to the qigong master and the surgeon.

This was the 10th thyroidectomy in a little over a month in which anesthesia with qigong was administered by Lin Housheng from the Shanghai Traditional Chinese Medicine Research Institute. Of these 10 operations, the results of nine were rated as "excellent," according to the standards set for acupuncture anesthesia, and the remaining one was classified "grade 3" because 10 ml of local anesthetic had to be used. Eight of the nine "excellent" operations were aided with the use of 50 mg of dolantin (this dosage is permissible in acupuncture anesthesia) while the remaining one was performed without any drugs.

In addition, Lin had helped in three successful subtotal gastrectomies.

He Learned Qigong Early

Lin, 41, hails from Fuqing County, Fujian Province. A sports lover since childhood, he began practicing qigong when he was in junior middle school. After finishing a three-year course he was recommended to the wushu department of the Shanghai Physical Culture Institute.

Upon graduation in 1964 he was given a job at the local sports research institute. In 1968, after long years of qigong practice, he felt that something was ejecting from the center of his palm when he was doing the qigong exercises. By way of experiment he began to apply this "something" to the treatment of stomach ulcers, high blood pressure, protrusion of lumbar vertebra and other chronic ailments.

To his surprise, he found it really helped! The thing that did the miraculous work is waiqi, which was identified later as a kind of low-frequency modulated infrared radiation by scientists at the Shanghai Atomic Nucleus Research Institute of the Chinese Academy of Sciences. This discovery heightened Lin's confidence in curing ailments with qigong.

Using the waiqi released from his palm or fingers, Lin had later developed various ways of treatment. One method, called "qizhen" ("air needle"), consists in inserting a tiny needle into a certain acupuncture point and applying waiqi to the needle to accentuate twirls. The patient's muscles twitch as currents of heat penetrate into them.

That was how he cured Hu Deshun, a 28-year-old peasant from suburban Shanghai. Fracture of the first lumbar vertebra made Hu a paraplegic in September 1977, with incontinence of faeces and urine. Two years of treatment by both Western and traditional Chinese medicine was of no avail. His leg muscles became flabby and weak, and he barely managed to stand up with the help of crutches.

In April 1980 he came to the Shanghai Traditional Chinese Medicine Research Institute where he received qizhen treatment from Lin Housheng. Gradually his legs regained strength and by the second month he was cured of urinary incontinence and could walk a few steps without crutches.

In the course of treatment, Lin discovered the analgesic effect of waiqi and it was then that he started his research of qigong-induced anesthesia. His success is being studied and analyzed by scientific research institutes.

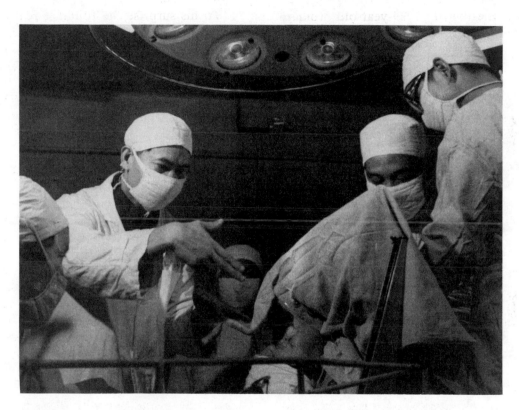

Qigong master Lin Housheng administering anaesthesia for a surgical operation at the Shanghai No. 8 People's Hospital.

HOW THE DAYAN QIGONG EXERCISE CURES

By LAO LIN

Reporter, New Sports Journal

During the last three years dayan qigong has been promoted on a mass scale in Beijing. Many people who used to suffer from poor health or chronic ailments have benefited from it. Here are just a few examples:

1. Qian Liangyu (female, age 49, teacher at the middle school attached to the People's University)

Began to suffer from hypertension in 1971. Medical treatment proved to be of no avail and her condition went from bad to worse until her blood pressure rose to 220/130 mmHg in 1978. Meanwhile, she fell victim to insomnia and could sleep no more than three or four hours every night even though she always took a sedative before going to bed. Prolonged illness reduced her to agony and despair.

After going in for dayan qigong, she could get along without taking medicine. Within a month her sleep had improved remarkably. Every day she went to bed after 9:30 p.m. and did not wake up until 5:30 the next morning. By the end of another month her blood pressure had dropped to a stable level of 150/90 mmHg. Her mental attitude had also greatly improved.

2. Jiang Hua (female, 54, worker at Beijing No. 798 Plant)

Suffered from chronic hepatitis for over 20 years. Troubled by insomnia as well. Hb:6g. Ate only 2-3 liang, or 100-150 g., of staple food a day. Forced to retire because of illness.

After a few weeks of dayan qigong practice, she felt much better and could consume 100-150 g. of staple food per meal. Her sleep had also improved.

Hb was increased to 9 g. within a month and 12.7 g. within three months. Liver function was restored to normal in four months.

3. Shao Xiu-e (female, 51, administrative cadre at the Beijing Boiler Plant)

Case history:

a. Pyelonephritis — RBC found in urine; edema.

b. Sequelae of brain thrombus — numbness in the limbs.

After three months of dayan qigong exercise, she felt stronger and light of foot. Results in repeated routine urine tests were normal. Numbness in limbs and edema had disappeared. Waist measurement had decreased from 86 cm to 80 cm.

4. Fan Jingzhong (male, 49, administrator at the No. 502 Research Institute of the Ministry of Astronautics Industry)

Case history:

a. Heart disease — arrhythmia.

b. Rheumatoid disease — lumbago which made movement difficult. Back of each hand was covered with large, black flecks attributable to old age.

After two months of dayan qigong practice, the heart problem was noticeably alleviated and the patient was able to exercise self-control when he did not feel well. For two years now there has been no relapse. Lumbago has also become much less intense. The patient can now move about easily and can even bend his waist. The flecks on his hands have become lighter in color and less protruding than before.

5. Xie Huanzhang (male, 64, professor at Beijing Industrial College)

Has been suffering from hypertension for 11 years, his blood pressure reaching 200/120 mmHg at one time. Also troubled by constipation. Blood pressure dropped to a stable level of 140/70 mmHg after two months' dayan qigong practice, during which time no medicine was taken. Constipation was also assuaged.

6. Wang Shangrui (male, 74, retired worker)

Suffered from lumbago for many years. After two months' dayan qigong practice, his appetite has increased, he can sleep very well and he no longer feels any pain in the lumbar region. His eyesight and hearing have also markedly improved. He can now read without wearing glasses and can hear the clicking sound of a watch placed behind his ears. He feels more energetic than ever.

POSTSCRIPT

In practicing the exercises in this book, you are working with some valuable Oriental concepts. One is the idea that the body and mind are an organic whole and should be developed together. Another is the idea of naturalness in mind and movement.

These concepts help to bring the body and mind into a natural harmony through relaxed but disciplined effort. Learning that from these exercises is learning a lot.

Aside from the obvious physical and emotional benefits that can be obtained from qigong practice, these exercises also offer an unique opportunity to improve understanding between the people of the West and the Chinese people. In a world where misunderstanding seems to be the rule rather than the exception, such an effort toward mutual understanding becomes increasingly valuable.

By making these exercises available outside of China, the Chinese people have taken the first step. It is really up to us to follow through on what they have made available, if only for our own individual benefit. But, hopefully, a broader and deeper fellowship will also develop.

We learn by doing. Your first efforts to learn these exercises may have seemed awkward. But you will find them easier and more enjoyable as you learn more. It is like learning a language. Fluency increases with practice. Your appetite for them will also grow with your confidence. But even the difficulty you may encounter is part of the experience we can share.

The case histories in the book show that the benefits were usually obtained through a strong effort over a period of time, often by people desperately ill.

Being moderately healthy should make perseverance that much easier and provide the potential for making more substantial progress. It is surely wise to place a high value on your own effort and perseverance.

Equally important and satisfying is continually cultivating the attitude of joyful play, which qigong helps to create.

If you can learn and practice with a sense of joy and a feeling that the exercises are not work but a natural kind of play, then you are beginning to capture their spirit. You will then certainly reap more of their benefits.

Marvin Smalheiser
Publisher
Wayfarer Publications

GLOSSARY

Baduanjin: A fitness exercise that literally means "beautiful eight sections brocade."

Dantian: An important acupuncture point and energy center located 5 cm below the navel. It is used to center the mind and body in many Oriental disciplines for health, meditation, fitness, and martial arts.

Daoyin: An ancient Chinese health-building exercise that combines regulated breathing with body movements. They were first recorded over 2,000 years ago.

Jingluo: Passages or meridians in the body, along which the acupuncture points are distributed and the qi flows.

Qi: The vital energy of the body. Qigong exercises amplify and balance the vital energy of the body.

Roc: A mythical bird of great size and strength believed to live in the Indian ocan.

Shaolin School: A famous martial art style developed at the famous Shaolin Temple in central China.

Taiji School: Taijiquan (T'ai Chi Ch'uan) is an ancient Chinese exercise and internal martial art beneficial to health and practiced by many millions of Chinese.

Yuan Qi: The original energy of the body.

Yijinjing: An ancient Chinese exercise for limbering the tendons.

Waiqi: Outflowing energy, or qi, that is projected by qigong experts, usually from their palms and which they use for healing.

Wuqin Qigong: A qigong exercise devised by a famous Chinese physician, Hua Tuo (?-203 A.D.). It is based on the movements of five animals: the ape, deer, tiger, bear, and bird.

Xingyi School: A Chinese style of martial arts that is one of the leading internal systems.

NOTES